over 130 recipes plus
nutrition and lifestyle advice

easy

wheat, egg and
milk-free cooking

rita greer

Thorsons

Thorsons

An Imprint of HarperCollins*Publishers*

77–85 Fulham Palace Road,

Hammersmith, London W6 8JB

The Thorsons website address is www.thorsons.com

First published by Thorsons 1984 as
Wheat, Milk & Egg-Free Cooking
Second edition 1989
Third edition 1995
This edition revised and updated 2001

10 9 8 7 6 5 4 3 2 1

A catalogue record for this book
is available from the British Library

ISBN 0 00 710317 4

**Printed and bound in Great Britain by
Martins the Printers Limited, Berwick upon Tweed**

contents

introduction

Wheat, milk and eggs are probably the three most common allergens (allergy-causing agents) in the Western diet today. They are 'staples' and are eaten every day by most of us in some form. While some people may be allergic to just one of these items, others less fortunate may be allergic to all three. As they play such an important part in the structure of our diet, a food regime which excludes them needs to be carefully balanced to replace their valuable nutrients.

The author has had personal and practical experience of catering for a special diet which cuts out wheat, milk and eggs, and the results of her research in the form of information and recipes has proved to be a lifeline for people on similar diets. This book gives a broad outline of the problem of cooking without these foods, and it offers practical advice, including a wide range of recipes, on how to cope with what may at first appear to be an impossible diet to follow.

wheat, milk and eggs

wheat

For most people wheat is a wonderful food! It is cheap, easy to grow and harvest, is highly nutritious and extremely versatile, keeps well and tastes good. One of its most interesting qualities is that when liquid is added to wheat flour it will make a very elastic dough that can be shaped and baked. It will also thicken, make smooth and bind other ingredients. We eat wheat mainly in the form of bread and other bakery products. It is also widely used in a variety of products from instant desserts to Communion wafers.

If you see one of the following items listed as an ingredient in a manufactured food, then it may well contain wheat and should be avoided.

cracked wheat	wheat flakes
durum wheat	wheat flour
kibbled wheat	wheat germ (and oil)
semolina	wheat protein
wheat	wheat starch
wheat berries	wheatmeal
wheat bran	wholegrain wheat

Any food that lists one or more of the following ingredients on the label may contain wheat:

binder	MSG (monosodium glutamate),
cereal	often made from wheat starch
cereal protein	rusk
corn	special edible starch
cornstarch (UK)	starch
flour	thickener
food starch	thickening
modified starch	vegetable protein

contamination by wheat

Rye, barley, oats and rice are traditionally stored, milled and packed in the same factories and mills as wheat. Contamination is inevitable, as in any flour mill wheat dust is everywhere – all over the machinery, on all ledges and surfaces, on the workers and in the air. So, while it would seem to be the obvious choice to use rye, barley, oats and rice flour on a wheat-free diet the contamination problem has made this difficult for some. There is also the point to be considered that rye, barley, oats and rice are not as versatile as wheat for baking, and usually they need to be combined with wheat flour for best results. Oats can be used on their own in a limited way, but appear in the shops as 'rolled oats' and 'oatmeal' and not as a flour. Oats have an individual taste and are not as bland as wheat.

A **very** allergic person would be wise not to use rye, barley or rice flour, oats or oatmeal because of the risk of wheat contamination. It is possible to buy ground rice that is guaranteed non-contaminated, but not rice flour. The **less** allergic person may be able to tolerate the wheat contamination in ordinary milled rye, barley, oats and rice. However, a return of symptoms may mean a stricter approach is necessary, and most people will probably feel it is not worth the risk, preferring a 100-per-cent wheat-free diet to a low-wheat diet.

contamination in the home

One of the problems of wheat-free baking is that contamination of wheat-free foods and ingredients can occur easily if care is not taken to avoid the problem. The main culprit will be wheat flour which is inclined to be dusty and easily becomes airborne. Wheat may also be present on tins and utensils and this too can lead to contamination. Most people on a wheat-free diet prefer to keep one set of utensils and baking tins etc., just for wheat-free cooking. Wheat flour under the fingernails, wheat flour on overalls or apron can also be a source of contamination. An electric toaster which is used for both wheat bread and wheat-free bread can again be a problem as the crumbs from both kinds of bread accumulate in the bottom. A way round this is to use the grill for toasting wheat-free bread and the toaster for ordinary bread.

For someone who is acutely allergic to wheat a separate set of utensils is a must. Otherwise be scrupulously clean and use the same utensils etc., for both types of baking/cooking.

what wheat provides

Basically wheat contributes carbohydrate, protein, vitamins (especially from the B group), minerals (especially iron) and cereal fibre to the diet. In the average diet wheat can provide up to one sixth of the daily intake of protein, more often than not in the form of bread.

To replace wheat in the diet other foods can be used, e.g. protein is readily available in meat and fish. The B-group vitamins can be supplemented by Brewer's Yeast or by vitamin tablets. Many previously bought ready-made foods will need to be made at home, such as bread, cakes, biscuits, etc. If wheat bran has previously been used in the diet, other types of fibre will have to be substituted such as rice bran or soya bran.

what to avoid

The following other products must not be consumed or used in wheat-free cooking *unless you are sure they do not contain any wheat:*

Baked beans in tomato sauce

Baking powder

Batter mixes

Bedtime drinks

Biscuits and biscuit mixes

Blancmange powders

Breadcrumbs

Breakfast cereals

Cakes and cake mixes

Cereals

Chocolate (cheap brands)

Chutney

Cocoa

Coffee (instant)

Communion wafers

Corned beef

Cornflour (cornstarch)

Cream (non-dairy)

Crispbreads

Crumble topping

Curry powder

Custard (powder or
    ready-made tinned)

Desserts and instant
    puddings

Drinking Chocolate

Gravy powder and mixes

Ice creams

Macaroni

Stuffings

Mayonnaise

Mustard

Oat porridge (instant)

Pancake mixes, pancakes

Pastas

Pastry mixes

Pickles

Pie fillings

Salad dressings

Sandwich spreads

Fish in coatings

Sauces

Sausages

Soups (tins and packets)

Soy sauce

Spaghetti

Sprouted grains

Stock cubes

Sweets

Yogurt (fruit flavours)

milk

Milk features in our diet in many forms – butter, cream, cheese and yogurt, or as a drink in various ways. In the Western world, dairy farming is an extremely important industry and milk is plentiful and cheap. It is not unusual for adults to drink at least ½ litre (1 pint) per day and children more.

Milk is added to products to enrich them. Components of milk can also be used in manufacturing. Lactose (milk sugar) is widely used as a filler in the manufacture of pharmaceuticals. Caseinate (milk protein) is valuable as an enricher and is used to increase the nutritional value of slimming products and cheeses. Whey is used in the manufacture of margarines usually to make them creamy.

If you see any of the following items listed as an ingredient in a food it will not be milk-free:

Albumin

Calcium *

Casein *

Curds

Iron *

Lactic acid

Lactose (milk sugar)

Magnesium *

Milk

Milk protein

Milk solids

Potassium *

Sodium *

Whey

Zinc *

* caseinates

The following products should not be used in milk-free cooking *unless you are sure they do not contain milk:*

Bakery foods, such as
   cakes, buns, pastries
   and biscuits
Baking powder
Batter mixes
Butter and cream sauces
Butter/butter-like spreads
Cake mixes
Cake toppings
Cheeses (all kinds)
Chocolate
Chocolate, cocoa and other
   milk-based drinks
Condensed milk
Cream
Creamed foods
Custard (ready-made)
Dried milk
Evaporated milk

Ice cream
Instant desserts
Instant pudding mixes
Junket
Margarine
Mashed potato
Pancake and waffle
   mixes
Pastry
Salad dressings
Scrambled eggs
Skimmed milk
Slimming foods
Soups
Spreads
Sweets
Whole milk
Yogurt
Yorkshire pudding

what milk provides

Milk contributes carbohydrate, fat, protein, calcium, iron, Vitamin A, Vitamin B_2, and other vitamins and minerals to our diet. It is a liquid food and therefore easy to add to food intake, and it will also mix into other foods easily. To replace milk in the diet other carbohydrate, fat and protein foods such as potatoes, cooking oil, meat and fish can be substituted. Cod liver oil or fish oils will provide Vitamin A. For Vitamin B_2 (Riboflavin) liver is a good source. Calcium can be replaced by Calcium gluconate, Dolomite, B_{13} Calcium (calcium orotate) or bonemeal taken as a supplement. This calcium supplementation is especially important in children's diets as it is necessary for the growth of strong bones, teeth and nails.

contamination in the home

Scrupulous cleanliness is essential to avoid contamination, with extra care during washing up. Avoid using the same spoon to stir a non-milk drink when everyone else in the family is having a drink containing milk. This kind of attitude should not be considered to be fussy – merely careful.

Generally speaking, milk contamination is less of a hazard than wheat, as milk is usually liquid. Do be careful with dried milk before you mix it with water as it can be dusty and has a nasty habit of sticking to the spoon.

eggs

Eggs provide a cheap form of food which is very nutritious. Because of the two parts of an egg, the protein-rich white (albumen) and the fat-rich yolk, its versatility in cooking is quite staggering. In particular the white can be aerated to make meringue, and beaten into other foods to bind them together. The yolk can be used to make emulsions such as mayonnaise.

If you see any of the following items listed as an ingredient in a manufactured food it means that egg has been used in its production, and it should therefore be avoided:

Albumen	Egg yolk
Dried egg	Fresh egg
Egg	Lecithin (unless from soya)
Egg glaze	Meringues
Egg lecithin	Whole egg
Egg white	

The following must not be used in egg-free cooking, *unless you are sure they do not contain egg*:

Batter mixes	Meat balls
Batter-coated foods	Quiche
(such as fish fingers)	Salad cream
Bedtime drinks	Sauces
Beefburgers	Scotch egg
Custard	Spaghetti and pastas
Fish cakes	Sponge and cake mixes
Ice cream	

what eggs provide

Eggs contribute protein and fat, calcium, iron, Vitamin A and other vitamins and minerals. They can be replaced in the diet with more meat and fish, but as an aid to cooking they are irreplaceable. You may come across so-called 'egg replacers' while shopping, but a glance at the ingredients list on the pack will reveal that they are largely starch in composition and nutritionally nothing like an egg. However, binders such as grated apple and pectin can be incorporated into foods so that they don't fall into crumbs. Oils can be substituted for egg yolks to make mayonnaise, but they will not have the yellow colouring of egg yolk.

contamination in the home

Extra care is required during cleaning of utensils, cutlery, etc., to avoid contamination. In particular, forks can trap cooked egg between the prongs. Egg white has a very strong tendency to attach itself to utensils, baking sheets, etc. If very stubborn it should be scraped off with a knife. As with wheat and milk contamination the answer to egg contamination is scrupulous cleanliness and great care.

are you allergic?

An allergy, intolerance or sensitivity to wheat, milk or eggs may manifest itself in one or more symptoms. It is difficult to be specific about what is causing the symptoms as they can also be caused by other factors. **People with persistent symptoms should consult their medical practitioner and not try to diagnose and treat themselves.**

physical symptoms

head

Feeling dizzy or faint, headaches, migraine, heavy feeling.

eyes

Watery, itchy, red, swollen, tired, sore, blurred vision, heavy feeling in eyelids.

nose

Runny nose, sneezing, itching, burning, excessive mucus, blocked nose, sinusitis.

ears

Ringing in the ears, soreness, loss of hearing, earache, burning sensations, itching.

throat and mouth

Soreness, sore gums, swollen tongue, mouth ulcers, loss of taste, hoarseness, cough, choking fits, itching of the roof of the mouth, bad breath.

heart and lungs

Chest pains, palpitations, rapid heartbeat, asthma, chest congestion, tightness across chest, shallow breathing, excessive sighing, breathlessness, catarrh.

gastro-intestinal

Nausea, vomiting, stomach cramps, diarrhoea, constipation, swollen stomach, bloated feeling after eating, flatulence, feeling 'full up' long after meals, stomach pains, poor appetite, cravings for foods, dyspepsia.

skin

Rashes, hives, inexplicable bruises, easily marked skin, eczema, excessively pale colour, dermatitis, itching, soreness, redness, sores, acne.

other physical symptoms

Weakness, cramp, cold hands and feet, flushing, shivering fits, trembling, aches and pains in the joints, swelling of the limbs, aches and pains in the muscles, swelling of the face, hands, feet, ankles, constant feeling of hunger, gorging with food, oedema, obesity.

behavioural and psychological symptoms

Nervousness, anxiety, panic attacks, depression, apathy, irritability, day-dreaming, confusion, restlessness, poor concentration, mood swings, aggression, unreasonable giggling or weeping, speech difficulties, couldn't-care-less attitude, general feeling of misery, excessive sleeping, hyperactivity, insomnia.

planning a diet without wheat, milk and eggs

Before the miseries set in, here is a list of the foods that you **can** eat:

the *yes* list – basic wheat-free, milk-free and egg-free foods

- Plain, fresh meat – all kinds
- Bacon
- Ham – without breadcrumb coating
- Plain, fresh, frozen or canned fish (in water) – all kinds
- All fresh vegetables
- All fresh fruit
- Rice – preferably brown
- Ground rice
- Maize (corn), cornflour (cornstarch)
- Barley flour
- Millet flour
- Porridge oats
- Sesame seeds

- Chickpea (gram) flour
- Plain, fresh nuts
- Pure cooking oils, such as safflower, sunflower, extra virgin olive oil, soya and corn oils
- Pure honey
- Treacle, syrup and molasses
- All kinds of sugars and jams

Drinks:

- Tea without milk
- Coffee without milk
- Herb teas
- Wine – red, white or rosé made from fruit
- Brandies derived from fruit
- Sherry
- Port

other wheat-free, milk-free and egg-free foods

N.B. Where brand names are specified this indicates that other brands of the same product may be unsuitable.

- Baked beans *(Heinz)* in tomato sauce (check label)
- Soya flour
- Ground almonds
- Frozen, plain fish and shellfish
- Tamari-type wheat-free soy sauce *(see page 21)*
- Frozen, plain meat
- Curry powder (a brand which does not contain wheat flour)

- Yeast extract *(Marmite)*
- Rice bran, soya bran
- Soya milk (not to everyone's taste, but some people find it useful)
- Dairy-free margarine
- Split peas
- Dried beans
- Lentils
- Soya beans
- Gelatine

Many people find a new kind of diet extremely worrying, particularly if their basic knowledge of nutrition is not adequate to restructure their daily menus. To exclude wheat, milk and eggs from the food regime and still eat a balanced diet can be nutritionally disastrous if care is not taken over the following points.

The greatest danger lies in eating too little protein, fibre, vitamin A, iron and calcium. This can result in a rather alarming weight loss, constipation, lethargy and a feeling of being 'below par'. Such a situation is easily rectified by increasing the consumption of fish and meat, taking a new kind of fibre in the form of rice or soya bran, and supplementation of the diet with vitamin A, iron and calcium in capsule or tablet form. Alternatively, suitable foods that contain these last three substances can be eaten regularly:

Vitamin A – oily fish
Iron – curry powder, spinach, watercress, dates, pineapple, sultanas, cocoa, prunes, figs
Calcium – sardines, watercress, figs, rhubarb, almonds and other nuts

By eating a wide variety of raw or lightly cooked vegetables and other permitted foods, any other resulting deficiencies in vitamins and minerals can be made up.

Once the new diet is underway, some people may experience a craving for wheat, milk and eggs. This is not an unusual reaction and to cope with it best requires a little extra effort in the kitchen to make the new diet exciting, satisfying and nutritious.

a balanced diet

Nobody knows exactly what each person requires in the way of nutrients as no two people have the same dietary needs. Much depends on what kind of life the person leads, how much energy he or she expends, his or her age and sex.

The average Western diet has many faults – usually containing too much fat, sugar and salt and not enough fibre, fresh vegetables and fruit, because too many processed and 'junk' foods are consumed instead.

Try to balance the daily food intake in this way:

15 per cent milk-free margarine, nuts, seeds and oils
25 per cent fish and meat
45 per cent fresh fruit and vegetables
15 per cent special bakery items

Try to use plain, fresh foods and not processed ones to minimize problems. The food in a wheat-free, milk-free, egg-free diet is not balanced in the same way as in a diet where these are staples. Here are the basic food values in a wheat-free, milk-free, egg-free diet:

Protein – meat, fish, nuts
Fat – cooking oils, meat, fish, nuts and seeds
Carbohydrate – rice, potatoes, bananas, special bread and bakery items, sugar, honey
Fibre – soya bran, rice bran, root vegetables, dried fruits
Vitamins and minerals – fresh vegetables and fruit

Bear in mind the advice given at the beginning of this book on replacing the nutrients that will be missing by the exclusion of wheat, milk and eggs. If the need for a vitamin and mineral supplement is felt, remember that like the food, any tablets etc. should also be wheat, milk and egg-free. Check with your medical practitioner or pharmacist before purchasing.

eating out

Eating out can be a big problem. Most restaurants will be totally unable to cope with a special diet of any description. The safest choice on this particular diet is:

Melon (plain) or fresh grapefruit (plain)
Grilled steak (without gravy or sauce) with a green salad (without dressing); plain boiled
    potatoes or rice
Fresh fruit

Eating out in someone else's home can also be difficult. The majority of hosts/hostesses will not be able to cope with such a strict diet any more than a restaurant can. Many will be much relieved when you offer to bring your own food, saving them the trouble of preparing a separate menu and you the worry of eating the wrong things.

The easiest items to take are (for a three-course meal):

Special soup, hot, in a vacuum flask, ready to serve
Cold meat, salad and cold, sliced, boiled potatoes – take special dressing in a separate
    container – arrange on a plate and cover with plastic film until it is served
Fruit salad or fruit.

packed meals

If meals have to be eaten regularly away from home, packed meals are the answer. Try to balance the meals as you would those eaten at home. Avoid too many snack items which will give you too much carbohydrate.

The easiest items will be hot soup in a vacuum flask; cold meat or canned fish in oil or water; salad with dressing packed in a separate container; crispbreads, cold brown rice or cold potato and fresh fruit and/or a piece of special fruit cake/biscuits. Wide-necked vacuum flasks can be used to take hot meals such as curry and brown rice.

holidays

Holidays are really just an extension of the eating-out problem. Self-catering holidays, although they are more work, certainly are less worry. Some items such as fruit cake and special bread can be made in advance and taken on holiday to use as required. Any special items that you may have difficulty in obtaining when you get to your destination, such as milk-free margarine, wheat-free soy sauce, special supplements, special brands, etc. must be taken as luggage. With a few exceptions, fresh vegetables, fruit, meat and fish are obtainable everywhere the world over.

Obviously, more planning is needed than for an ordinary holiday and more luggage is needed too. However, there is no reason why holidays away from home shouldn't be enjoyed. If you are travelling by plane take your own packed meal to eat during the flight. If going by car take a picnic, and so on.

If you are on a diet that will make you healthier then that diet is an enviable one. With a little effort your food can be enviable too.

pepper

A word of warning about the use of pepper. It is common practice in commercial catering to add wheat flour to ground white pepper to 'stretch' this expensive commodity. It is therefore a good practice to use only freshly ground black pepper when you are eating out. It is possible to buy pocket-sized miniature pepper grinders to solve this very problem.

stock

Most stock cubes, gravy powders and liquid stocks contain wheat. Those with monosodium glutamate (MSG) should be avoided as MSG can be derived from wheat. Soy sauces are traditionally made with soya beans and wheat but there is one kind which is made from soya beans and **rice.** This kind is the **Tamari** type. You are most likely to find it in health stores. Phone around your local health stores to find stockists. It keeps for years so don't be afraid to buy several bottles at a time. Note: Tamari is not a brand name. It refers to a special type of wheat-free soy sauce.

margarine

Most supermarkets stock a 'dairy-free' margarine which will be milk-free. However, take care it does not contain wheat germ oil (check labels).

spices

Use **pure** spices and mixtures of spices, e.g. curry powder, without 'fillers' or extenders. More expensive known brands are safest.

wheat, milk and egg-free menus

A special diet doesn't have to be a miserable, restricted regime. Here is an eight-day example using recipes from this book.

day one

Breakfast – Savoury Breakfast Cakes

Lunch – Mixed Salad with a slice of cold beef or ham without breadcrumbs; Special Crispbread; fruit

Tea – Fruit Cake

Dinner – Cauliflower Soup; Liver with Orange and Bacon, greens, root vegetables, mashed potato, gravy; Stuffed Baked Fruit

Snacks – Fruit and nuts, banana

day two

Breakfast – Suitable baked beans on special toast, unsweetened fruit juice

Lunch – Mixed green salad with tinned fish (in oil), mashed potato

Tea – Special Fruit Cake

Dinner – Fresh Pea Soup; Pork Chop with Apple Salad, jacket potato with special milk-free, wheat-free margarine; Fruit Dessert

Snacks – Ginger Thins, nuts

day three

Breakfast – Small Muesli; grilled bacon and mushrooms

Lunch – Lentil Soup, special bread (toasted) and milk-free margarine; Fruit Salad

Tea – Fruit Salad Cake

Dinner – Liver Pâté with special toast; Prawns Italian with brown rice, large green salad; orange

Snacks – Fruit and nuts, Digestive Biscuits

day four

Breakfast – Kedgeree

Lunch – Cold meat (chicken) and salad with mashed potato; fresh fruit

Tea – Fruit Salad Cake

Dinner – Beef Casserole with Orange, jacket potato, spinach or greens; Baked Fruit

Snacks – Crispbreads, special milk-free, wheat-free margarine and raw sugar jam (jelly)

day five

Breakfast – Cold meat and fried potatoes

Lunch – Fresh Pea Soup, Sippets; jacket potato with special milk-free margarine

Tea – Salad and mashed potato

Dinner – Tomato Starter; Fish Casserole, green vegetables, boiled brown rice; Stewed Fruit

Snacks – Fresh fruit

day six

Breakfast – Bubble and Squeak with grilled bacon

Lunch – Fish and Chips

Tea – Spiced Fruit Cookies

Dinner – Grapefruit; Chicken Curry with brown rice and green salad; Poppadoms; fresh
fruit or Fruit Salad

Snacks – Bananas, nuts

day seven

Breakfast – Savoury Breakfast Cakes

Lunch – Cold fish, mixed salad, mashed potato; fruit

Tea – Special toast, special milk-free, wheat-free margarine and raw sugar jam (jelly)

Dinner – Lemon Chicken, boiled brown rice, stir-fry vegetables with greens; Fruit Salad
(with lychees if in season)

Snacks – Spiced Fruit Cookies

day eight

Breakfast – Fruit Pancakes

Lunch – Roast lamb, mint sauce, roast potatoes, green vegetables; Fried Bananas

Tea – Special bread or Fruit Loaf and milk-free, wheat-free margarine; mixed salad with
cold fish (tinned); special cake (from *Teas and Treats* section)

Snacks – Party Almonds, Special Cheese and Crispbreads

(See back of book for lists of suggestions for meals.)

children on a special diet

Children on a very restricted diet, such as wheat, milk and egg free, need special care and understanding because being different does not make a child feel good. A sense of belonging to a group can be helped by sharing food with friends. For example, give your child a bag of home-made savoury snack nibbles to share (see page 72); these are more than a match for commercial versions. Meals must be attractive, nutritious and tasty. Sharing family meals some days is good for the young special dieter and something of a relief for the cook.

For children to grow and develop properly, they need to eat regularly, and older children may need more food than adults. Food is very important to a child. As adults, we can lose sight of this as we are more geared to watching our waistlines.

The temptation to consume inappropriate food is a constant problem. Relatives and friends who don't understand the special diet are apt to offer the wrong food as a 'kindness'. Mostly this will be in the form of snack foods, drinks and confectionery. The child should be taught how to handle the situation and to know which foods are acceptable and which are not. That way the child gains control of the situation and not the misinformed relatives or friends.

Encourage children to eat fresh fruit such as apples and bananas. Plain toasted nuts are another good snack. Toast your own plain nuts at home and keep them in a jar.

Parents of school children on a strict diet should make sure the head teacher knows about the situation. A special packed lunch is safer and less of a worry than expecting the school meals service to cope. Encourage children to be responsible for themselves. Any friend's mum who panics about coping with a special diet will be delighted when the special food turns up with the guest.

Always insist to the child that they are 'special' and that is why they need to be on a special diet. This is much more positive than taking the attitude that the child is a nuisance due to the difficulties of the diet.

Cravings for the very foods which have to be avoided are often the cause of the diet being broken. The answer to this is to provide good substitutes. The recipes in this book have been designed with this in mind.

shopping and the store cupboard

You will find that a special diet needs special shopping, and unless you plan sensibly this could mean extra hours of trekking round the shops without much success. Your best friend in this project could turn out to be the telephone as this will save a tremendous amount of time and energy. Items which you cannot obtain easily may have to be bought by mail order. However you obtain these special foods, it is common sense to build up a stock of them in your store cupboard.

Although friends may at first offer assistance with your special shopping, they usually become less anxious to help as it starts to become a weekly burden. Usually small shops are more helpful than large stores and will order in say a dozen bottles of a particular kind of soy sauce for you providing you will buy all 12 at once. Although a more expensive way of shopping is to order items by mail it is relatively effortless and they can be delivered right to your door. Usually the more you buy the cheaper it works out, and some firms offer free delivery over a certain amount.

store cupboard ingredients and where to buy them

Here is a list of items that could form the basis of a sensible store cupboard, ones you would be wise not to run out of:

Item	Buy at
Tinned fish in oil or water (not sauce) – sardines, tuna, salmon	Supermarket
Wheat-free (Tamari-type) soy sauce	Health Store
Baked beans in tomato sauce (Heinz UK) (check label)	Supermarket
Rice (preferably brown)	Supermarket or Health Store
Ground rice	Supermarket or Health Store
Soya flour	Health Store
Oatmeal/Porridge oats	Supermarket or Health Store
Maize flour/cornflour (make sure of a wheat-free brand)	Health Store or Supermarket
Potato flour (farina)	Health Store
Vinegar (wine or cider)	Supermarket or Health Store
Yeast	Supermarket or Health Store
Gelatine	Supermarket
Brown sugar (raw cane)	Health Store or Supermarket
Millet flour	Health Store
Chickpea flour	Health Store
Barley flour	Helath Store
Sesame seeds	Supermarket or Health Store
Treacle/molasses	Supermarket or Health Store
Salt (sea salt)	Health Store or Supermarket
Peppercorns (black)	Supermarket
Fruit juices (tinned)	Supermarket
Spices (make sure brands are wheat-free)	Supermarket

Curry powder (make sure of a wheat-free brand)	Supermarket
Dried herbs	Health Store or Supermarket
Milk-free margarine	Supermarket or Health Store
Herb teas	Supermarket or Health Store

The shop you will use most on this diet is the supermarket (or the butcher, fishmonger and greengrocer), so most of your shopping should be quite easy.

If you are looking for a wheat-free, milk-free margarine, read ingredients labels carefully, as wheatgerm oil is sometimes added to margarine for its vitamin E content. Most margarines contain whey, which is a milk by-product, but there are now milk-free margarines available. These are labelled 'dairy-free'. Kosher (Jewish) margarines are dairy-free.

In Mediterranean countries most people do not use margarine, preferring instead to drizzle olive oil on to bread and over hot vegetables. Although a little butter is eaten sometimes, olive oil is the main fat in the diet. It is by far the healthiest, particularly extra virgin, cold-pressed olive oil, so it is worth considering as an alternative to margarine and butter. Every supermarket has a selection so there should be no difficulty obtaining it.

special baking powder

Make your own baking powder (raising powder) and make sure that it does not contain wheat-flour or any milk by-product such as lactose.

7g/¼oz/2 tsp	**potassium bicarbonate**
115g/4¾oz/¾ cup	**potato flour/farina**

Mix and store in a screwtop jar. Use as required. Potassium bicarbonate can be bought at chemists.

local help

It may be worth finding out if there is a local allergy group which may be able to supply the names and addresses of useful suppliers of specialized foods and products. They may also be able to supply you with information about mail-order companies.

starting quickly with wheat, milk and egg-free

As it will take a few days or perhaps even a few weeks, depending where you live, to get organized with a new eating regime, here are some suggestions for menus using readily available ingredients. This should enable you to begin the new diet immediately instead of waiting until you have bought all the special foods you might need.

breakfasts

Savoury Breakfast Cakes (*see page 43*).
or Muesli with rice base (*see pages 46*).
or 2 slices grilled back bacon, grilled tomatoes and fried potato (pre-cooked the day before).
Drinks: Pure fruit juice, black coffee or tea with lemon.

mid-morning

Drinks: Black coffee or tea with lemon.
Few sultanas (golden seedless raisins) or raisins and shelled almonds.

lunch

Fish canned in oil or water – sardines, tuna or salmon, plus baked jacket potato, large mixed salad of lettuce, cucumber, grated carrot, tomato, dressed with wine vinegar, sunflower oil, a sprinkle of raw cane sugar and sea salt and freshly ground black pepper.
Follow with an apple or pear.
Drink: Water.

mid-afternoon

Drinks: Black coffee, lemon or herb tea.
1 banana or apple, or other fresh fruit in season.

dinner

Fruit juice followed by grilled lamb or pork chop or grilled steak with lightly cooked green vegetables and plain boiled potatoes or rice. No gravy except the vegetable juices.
Alternatively: use the Beef Casserole with Orange recipe (*see page 107*) or Good Old Fashioned Stew (*see page 114*).
End the meal with a fresh fruit salad.

If you feel hungry at any time during the day eat raisins and plain shelled nuts. If you are not used to black coffee or lemon tea, drink just plain water.

wheat, milk and egg-free basics

There are some foods or special items you will wish to eat or use every day and at any time of the day, perhaps even at every meal. Here are the basic recipes you will need for these:

staples

Without wheat, making bread can be difficult. It is worth trying suitable types of crispbread (*see Note to Cooks on page 37*) to see if they can be tolerated. Look at the ingredients list on the packet or carton and check with the lists given in this book to see if they are wheat-free, milk-free and egg-free.

Millet flour, barley flour, porridge oats and gram (chickpea) flour are useful in small amounts as part of a wheat-free flour blend.

active dried yeast

This is not mixed into the flour like Easyblend (instant) yeast. It needs to be mixed with warm water and allowed to swell before adding to the flour. If you are using this type of yeast, take some of the water from the recipe, warm it and sprinkle in the yeast with the sugar. Leave it in a warm place until frothy, then stir and add to the flour with the rest of the liquid.

fast-action instant yeast

This kind of yeast has additives to make it work more quickly. Check the ingredients list to see it does not contain any wheat, milk or egg in any form.

homemade pectin

Without enough gluten, baking disintegrates into a pile of crumbs. Pectin from apples, a replacement for gluten, can be made using something usually thrown in the bin. The liquid pectin available from stores and pharmacies is really for setting jam and not suitable for breadmaking.

Whenever you peel a cooking apple, save the peelings. Wrap in food film and immediately put into the freezer until required.

Put the peel from a medium cooking apple into a small saucepan with 1 cupful of water and bring to the boil. Cook without covering for up to 15 minutes, until the liquid has reduced by three-quarters. Save the strainings as you pour through a wire mesh sieve, pressing the peelings with the back of a wooden spoon. Discard the skin and put the strainings to one side to cool. It will form a pale green liquid. This is rich in pectin.

wheat-free bread

This loaf does not need to be left to rise before baking as it will rise well in the oven.

makes one small loaf

120g/4oz/⅔ cup	**ground rice**
60g/2oz/½ cup	**barley flour**
30g/1oz	**oat flour**
¼ tsp	**salt**
1 level tsp	**sugar**
7g/¼oz	**instant yeast**
1 tbs	**sunflower oil**
2 tbs	**homemade pectin** *(see page 34)*
200ml/7fl oz/¾ cup	**lukewarm water**
	sesame seeds for topping

1   Preheat oven to 350°F/180°C/gas mark 4.
2   Grease a 500g/1lb loaf tin.
3   Put the ground rice, flours, salt, sugar and yeast into a bowl. Mix well.
4   Add the pectin and water. Mix to a thick, creamy batter.
5   Turn into the prepared tin, sprinkle with sesame seeds and immediately put on the top shelf to bake for about 1 hour, until well-risen and golden with a cracked top.
6   Turn out onto a wire rack to cool as soon as it is baked. Do not cut until cold as the loaf needs to 'set'.
7   Eat freshly baked or the following day, toasted. Keep wrapped in food film to prevent the loaf from drying out.

note to cooks   To make oat flour, grind porridge oats in a coffee grinder (electric).

barley crispbreads

2 heaped tbs	**barley flour, plus extra for rolling out**
1 heaped tbs	**fine oatmeal**
pinch	**salt**
1 tsp	**sunflower or olive oil, plus extra for greasing**

1 Put the flour, oatmeal and salt into a bowl and mix well. Sprinkle in the oil and add enough water to mix by hand to a soft dough.

2 Dust the work surface with barley flour and roll out small pieces of dough very thinly. Trim neatly with a sharp knife if you wish.

3 Heat a griddle or heavy-based frying pan and grease with a little oil, using a wad of kitchen paper.

4 Use a spatula to place the crispbreads in the pan. Cook over a high heat for about 4 minutes, then turn over and cook the other side.

5 Cool on a wire rack and then store in an airtight container. Eat within a few days.

note to cooks Mass-produced crispbreads may all look exactly the same but home-made ones can be all shapes and sizes. So as not to waste any dough, roll pieces out and cook them whatever shape they are. This gives them personality!

rye crispbreads

If everyone around you is eating crusty wheat bread and feeling sorry for you, that is the time to produce these intriguing, paper-thin crispbreads.

makes five to six

2 tbs	**rye flour**
1 tbs	**barley flour**
6 tbs	**water**
	sunflower oil for greasing

1 Preheat the oven to 500°F/250°C/gas mark 9.
2 Mix together the flours and stir in the water, then beat to a smooth batter.
3 Lightly grease a baking (cookie) sheet with sunflower oil. Pour spoonfuls of the batter on to the baking (cookie) sheet and allow to spread into circles.
4 Bake on the top shelf of the oven for about 9 to 10 minutes, until crisp and golden. Cool on a wire rack and eat on the day of baking.

note to cooks   Although it is possible to buy crispbreads that appear to be wheat-free, wheat is often used as a cheap flour for dusting down in manufacture.

poppadoms

makes two

45g/1½oz	**ground rice**
15g/½oz	**gram (chickpea) flour**
15g/½oz	**cornflour (cornstarch)**
2 good pinches	**salt**
5 tbs	**cold water**
	sunflower oil for greasing

1 Preheat oven to 425°F/220°C/gas mark 7. Put in a baking sheet.
2 Put the first four (dry) ingredients into a basin. Mix well.
3 Add the water and mix to a thin batter.
4 Heat a heavy-based frying pan. Using kitchen paper, lightly grease with oil.
5 Pour in half the batter, tilting the pan to spread it out into a circle. Cook over a medium heat for about 3 minutes then loosen with a spatula and turn over to cook on the other side.
6 Make the second poppadom then put both on the hot baking sheet. Bake for about 10 minutes until crisp and crunchy.
7 Serve with curries.

note to cooks   The trick is to get the consistency of the batter thin enough to run in the pan. If left to stand, the batter will thicken up and should be thinned down with a little more water before using.

flatbread

Ideal for breakfast, tea or a snack.

makes three

30g/1oz	**barley flour**
60g/2oz/⅓ cup	**ground rice**
2 good pinches	**bicarbonate of soda**
3 good pinches	**cream of tartar**
1 level tsp	**caster sugar**
15g/½oz	**polyunsaturated margarine (milk-free)**
30g/1oz	**fresh mashed potato**

1 Preheat the oven to 425°F/220°C/gas mark 7.

2 Mix the first five (dry) ingredients in a bowl.

3 Rub in the margarine and then the mashed potato.

4 Stir in enough water to bind and mix by hand to a smooth, stiff dough.

5 Break the dough into 3 pieces. Shape each one into a round or square scone.

6 Place on a greased baking sheet and bake for 15 minutes on the top shelf until golden.

7 Cool on a wire rack and eat freshly baked, split and buttered or just broken into pieces.

barley oatcakes

Serve instead of wheat bread with soups or salads or spread with milk-free margarine and jam for a snack.

makes eight to ten plain biscuits

115g/4oz/⅔ cup	medium oatmeal
30g/1oz	barley flour
1 good pinch	bicarbonate of soda
¼ level tsp	salt
30g/1oz	polyunsaturated, milk-free margarine
1–2 tbs	boiling water
	more barley flour for rolling out

1 Preheat oven to 375°F/190°C/gas mark 5.
2 Mix the first four (dry) ingredients in a bowl.
3 Rub in the margarine.
4 Put in 1 tablespoon boiling water. Use a knife to stir the dough together, adding another tablespoon of boiling water if required. Mix to a soft, sticky dough.
5 Sprinkle the worktop with barley flour. Divide the dough in two. Roll out each piece thinly and cut into circles with a tumbler or cutter.
6 Use a spatula to lift onto a greased baking sheet. Bake until dried out and crisp on the top shelf for about 20 minutes.
7 Cool on a wire rack and store in an airtight container.

breakfasts

This is probably the greatest problem meal for a wheat-free, egg-free, milk-free dieter. With the traditional breakfast being egg based with wheat cereals and milk, other forms of protein must be used for this very important first meal of the day. As this section relies on simple dishes most come as suggestions and not recipes.

If sitting down to breakfast becomes a misery when you have to watch the rest of the family tucking in to all the things you are not allowed, take your breakfast on a tray, away from the table. Why not spoil yourself and have breakfast in bed?

If you like a large breakfast then fruit juice, fresh fruit or stewed fruit can be your starter. Follow with a protein dish such as grilled bacon, baked beans or cold meat. If you are still hungry, try a non-wheat cereal moistened with soya milk. Tea or coffee without milk and you should be well set up for the morning! (You will undoubtedly be able to buy at least one kind of wheat-free breakfast cereal at your local health store or supermarket, and soya milk too, if you don't mind it.)

bubble and squeak

To eat with cold meat or grilled bacon. This is a simple, traditional British dish. Chop left-over cooked greens and potato. Using a frying pan, cook in a little sunflower oil to prevent it sticking for 5 minutes each side over a medium heat. When brown on one side, turn over and brown on the other. Your finished dish should be a compressed flattish cake of vegetables, crisp and brown on the outside and soft in the middle.

savoury breakfast cakes

50g/2oz	cold, boiled potato
generous knob	milk-free margarine
50g/2oz	cold minced ham (without breadcrumb coating)
sprinkle	chopped parsley
	sea salt
	freshly ground black pepper
	vegetable oil for frying

1   Mash the potato with the margarine.

2   Put into a bowl and add the ham and parsley. Mix well.

3   Season to taste and shape into two round, flat cakes.

4   Heat a little oil in a frying pan.

5   Put in the savoury cakes and fry on both sides until browned, about 4 minutes on each side.

6   Serve hot with grilled tomatoes, fried mushrooms and/or wheat-free baked beans in tomato sauce.

note to cooks   Other kinds of meat can be used such as cold leftover beef or lamb from a joint. Bacon can be used too. Grill then chop into small pieces. Fish such as cold grilled haddock or cod (filleted) and canned salmon or tuna (in oil) will add variety. Drain off all the oil before flaking. If oatmeal can be eaten without ill-effects then the savoury cakes can be rolled in oatmeal before frying. This will give a crisper texture.

beans on fried bread

Fry slices of wheat-free bread in shallow hot oil until golden and crisp. Serve on a hot plate topped with wheat-free baked beans in tomato sauce, heated in a small saucepan. Grilled tomatoes, fried mushrooms and grilled bacon can be added to make the dish more substantial.

If the idea of fried bread does not appeal then try toasted wheat-free bread spread with milk-free margarine.

potato nest

For this you will need a shallow fireproof dish that will fit under the grill. Put a generous portion of cold mashed potato (make sure it was mashed with milk-free, wheat-free margarine) into the dish and flatten with a knife. Put under a medium grill for about 10 minutes when the top will be crisp and the potato heated right through. Make a well in the centre through to the bottom of the dish. Fill this with hot, wheat-free baked beans in tomato sauce and top with a sprinkle of chopped grilled bacon or ham. Serve on a plate, still in the fireproof dish.

kedgeree

Mix 2 or 3 tablespoonsful of cold, cooked brown rice with a chopped tomato, chopped ham, cold flaked fish, cooked peas or sweetcorn. Mix and season to taste. Heat a little oil in a frying pan and heat the mixture through. Serve on a hot plate. Freshly chopped parsley can also be added before serving. (Ham should be without breadcrumbs.)

whitebait

See section on Soups, Starters and Snacks for this recipe. Makes a good protein-high breakfast.

grilled fish

See section on Main Meals for this recipe. Serve with wheat-free bread and milk-free margarine.

cold meat with fried potato

Choose from cold roast beef or lamb cut off a joint, or ham without breadcrumb coating. Fry cold, boiled potatoes left over from the day before, in a little sunflower oil and serve with grilled tomatoes or wheat-free and milk-free tomato sauce.

muesli

For those people who cannot entertain the thought of a substantial breakfast a muesli might be the answer.

In a dish put 1 to 2 tablespoonsful of one of the suggested bases (*see below*). Sprinkle with 2 teaspoonsful of seeds. Add 1 piece of fresh fruit from the list and 1 heaped tablespoonful each of dried fruit and nuts. Sweeten with one of the suggested sweeteners and moisten with one of the liquids.

Bases: Cold cooked rice, rolled oats (if you can find a brand that you can tolerate without any ill-effects) or a non-wheat cereal.

Seeds: Sunflower seeds, sesame seeds.

Fresh fruit: Banana, apple, pear, nectarine, fresh plums, peach, strawberries, raspberries, sweet apricots and cherries, etc.

Dried fruit: Seedless raisins, sultanas (golden raisins), chopped dried apricots, peaches or stoned prunes.

Nuts: Any kind of plain nuts such as almonds, cashews, walnuts, hazelnuts, etc.

Sweeteners: Liquid honey, fructose (fruit sugar) or raw cane sugar.

Liquid: Spring water, soya milk (if liked), fruit juice.

toasted muesli

A delicious breakfast for the special dieter.

6	hazelnuts, cut into quarters
1 level tbs	cashew nut pieces
½ tbs	sesame seeds
1 heaped tbs	porridge oats
1 heaped tsp	demerara sugar
1	ripe banana, sliced
2	dried apricot halves, chopped
2	dates, stoned and chopped
	fresh apple juice to serve
2 tsp	runny honey

1   Cover the base of a sponge tin with the nuts, seeds, oats and sugar.
2   Put under a hot grill for a minute. Stir and continue to grill until golden brown. Put to one side to cool in the tin.
3   Slice the banana. Sprinkle with the dried fruit. Pour over a little apple juice and top with the toasted mixture.
4   Drizzle over the honey and serve.

note to cooks   Plain soya milk can be used instead of the apple juice. Apple can be used instead of the banana.

breakfast pizza

serves one

dough:

30g/1oz	millet flour
30g/1oz	cornflour (cornstarch)
60g/2oz/⅓ cup	ground rice
2 good pinches	bicarbonate of soda
3 good pinches	cream of tartar
1 good pinch	salt
30g/1oz	milk-free margarine
30g/1oz	(fresh) mashed potato
about 4 tbs	water

topping:

3	peeled plum tomatoes (canned)
2	lean rashers back bacon (fat removed)
1 medium	mushroom, chopped
1 tbs	sunflower oil
	salt and pepper to taste

1 Preheat oven to 425°F/220°C/gas mark 7.

2 Put the first six (dry) ingredients into a bowl and mix well.

3 Rub in the margarine and the mashed potato.

4 Add enough water to mix to a stiff paste. Knead into 1 ball of dough.

5 Place on a greased ovenproof plate and press out with the fingers to make a circle with a raised edge.

6 Cut the tomatoes up with kitchen scissors and spread over the pizza base.

7 Chop the bacon into small squares and scatter over the tomatoes.

8 Put the mushrooms into a small basin and spoon over the oil. Turn over to coat and spread over the pizza. Season to taste.

9 Bake on the top shelf for 15 minutes until the base is golden and the filling sizzling. Serve hot.

fruit pancakes

makes two

15g/½oz	**cornflour (cornstarch)**
15g/½oz	**barley flour**
60g/2oz/⅓ cup	**ground rice**
good pinch	**salt**
¼ level tsp	**caster sugar**
1 level tbs	**unsweetened stewed apple**
5 tbs	**water**
	sunflower oil for greasing
2 tbs	**sweetened stewed fruit**

1　Mix the first five (dry) ingredients in a bowl.

2　Stir in the stewed apple.

3　Add the water and beat to a thin batter.

4　Put a heavy-based frying pan on to heat. With a screw of kitchen paper and a little oil, grease the pan.

5　Pour half the batter into the centre of the pan. Tilt the pan to allow it to spread into a circle. Cook over a steady heat for about 3 minutes then turn over and cook on the other side.

6　Keep the pancake warm on a plate in the oven while you make the second one.

7　Spread each one with 2 tablespoons of sweetened stewed fruit and roll up.

8　Dust with caster sugar and serve hot.

note to cooks　The stewed apple should be beaten to make a smooth purée without any lumps.

stewed fruit suggestions

Apple; blackberry and apple; plum; plum and apple; summer fruits; greengages; apple and summer fruits; apple and blackberries; rhubarb; rhubarb and apple.

soups, starters and snacks

fresh pea soup

1 medium	onion, peeled and sliced
2 tsp	vegetable oil
400ml/¾ pint/2 cups	water
350g/¾ lb/2 cups	fresh peas, after shelling*
2 tsp	Tamari-type wheat-free soy sauce
	sea salt and freshly ground black pepper

1 Fry the onion in the oil for a few minutes, until transparent.
2 Add half the water, the peas and the soy sauce. Bring to the boil and simmer with the lid on for about 8 to 10 minutes.
3 Pour in the rest of the water, and liquidize.
4 Return to the saucepan, heat through, season to taste and serve hot.

* If fresh peas are not available, use frozen garden peas. Simmer for only 3 minutes after they have defrosted in the soup.

cock-a-leekie soup

serves four

1	chicken portion (e.g. leg), about 225g/8oz, skinned
1	leek, sliced
½	celery stalk, chopped
1 tbs	pearl barley
2 tsp	Tamari-type wheat-free soy sauce
	salt and freshly ground black pepper
1 heaped tsp	chopped fresh parsley

1 Put the chicken into a medium-sized pan and add water to cover. Bring to the boil, skimming off any scum that forms on the surface.
2 Add the leek, celery, barley, soy sauce and seasoning. Return to the boil, then reduce heat and simmer gently with the lid half on for about 1½ hours, topping up with boiling water if required.
3 Take out the chicken, cool a little and then take the meat off the bone. Shred and put back into the pan, then skim off the fat with a spoon.
4 Reheat and sprinkle with the parsley. Serve as a main meal with rice or a jacket potato.

lentil soup

125g/5oz/¾ cup	**lentils**
2 medium	**onions, peeled and sliced**
1 tbs	**vegetable oil**
1 medium	**potato, peeled and sliced thinly**
1 tbs	**Tamari-type wheat-free soy sauce**
½ litre/1 pint/2½ cups	**water**
	sea salt and freshly ground black pepper

1 Wash the lentils in a wire sieve and soak overnight in a large bowl with 850ml plus (1½ pints plus) of water (enough to cover).

2 Fry the onion in the oil for 3 to 4 minutes, using a large pan.

3 Add the potato, soy sauce, the strained lentils, the water and seasoning.

4 Bring to the boil and simmer for 40 minutes.

5 Remove from heat and allow to cool. Liquidize.

6 Serve hot with special bread sippets.

avocado soup

This is an unusual soup that must be served as soon as it is made or it will discolour. The final result is very creamy without adding milk or cream.

serves two

1 small	**onion, peeled and sliced finely**
1 tsp	**milk-free margarine**
1 medium	**avocado pear**
2 tsp	**Tamari-type wheat-free soy sauce**
¼ litre/½ pint/2½ cups	**water**
	sea salt
	freshly ground black pepper

1 Fry the onion in the margarine until transparent but not brown.
2 Peel the avocado and remove the stone.
3 Put fried onion and avocado flesh (cut into pieces) into the blender with the wheat-free soy sauce and water. Liquidize.
4 Return to the saucepan, heat and simmer for 3 or 4 minutes.
5 Season to taste and serve right away.

cauliflower soup

Make and serve immediately. A very creamy soup with a subtle flavour.

1 small	onion, peeled and sliced finely
1 tsp	milk-free margarine
½ small	cauliflower head
285ml/½ pint/2½ cups	water
1 tsp	cornflour/cornstarch
pinch	grated nutmeg
1 tsp	Tamari-type wheat-free soy sauce
	sea salt and freshly ground black pepper

1　Fry the onion in the margarine until transparent.

2　Cut the cauliflower into small pieces and put into the saucepan with half the water.

3　Bring to the boil and simmer for 5 minutes to soften. Remove from heat.

4　Mix the maize (cornstarch) with the remaining water and pour into the liquidizer goblet with the mixture from the saucepan.

5　Add the nutmeg and soy sauce.

6　Heat through and simmer for another 4 or 5 minutes while you stir.

7　Taste, season and serve hot, immediately.

note to cooks　The cauliflower should have creamy white curds and be nice and crisp. Avoid discoloured rubbery ones as they will be far from fresh.

french country soup

½ kilo/1 lb	**leeks, trimmed**
3	**carrots, trimmed**
1½ tbs	**vegetable oil**
½ kilo/1 lb	**potatoes, peeled**
¾ litre/1½ pints/3¾ cups	**water**
1 tbs	**Tamari-type wheat-free soy sauce**
	sea salt and freshly ground black pepper
1 heaped tbs	**fresh parsley, finely chopped**

1   Cut the leeks in half lengthways. Wash well and cut into small sections.

2   Chop the carrots into small pieces and fry in the oil with the leeks, while stirring, for about 5 minutes.

3   Add the potato, cut into thin slices and about two-thirds of the water. Also add the soy sauce, then bring to the boil and simmer with the lid on for about 20 to 25 minutes.

4   Remove from heat and add the rest of the water. Liquidize in a blender and return to saucepan. Taste and season.

5   Reheat and stir in the chopped parsley. Serve hot.

note to cooks   The potatoes make this a very filling soup. Serve to the whole family.

onion and potato soup

1 large	**onion, peeled and sliced thinly**
1 tbs	**sunflower oil**
1	**garlic clove, peeled and chopped**
2 medium	**potatoes, peeled and sliced**
400ml/¾ pint/2 cups	**cold water**
2 tsp	**Tamari-type wheat-free soy sauce**
	sea salt and freshly ground black pepper

1   Fry the onion in the oil for 3 or 4 minutes.

2   Crush in the garlic and stir.

3   Add the potato, half the water and the soy sauce. Heat through and simmer for about 10 to 12 minutes with the lid on.

4   Remove from heat, add the remaining water and liquidize in a blender.

5   Pour back into the saucepan and season to taste.

6   Serve hot.

optional   Sprinkle in a little freshly chopped parsley, just before serving.

mushroom and tomato soup

1 medium	**onion, peeled and sliced**
1 tbs	**vegetable oil**
100g/4oz/2 cups	**fresh mushrooms, washed and sliced**
400ml/¾ pint/2 cups	**tomato juice**
2 tsp	**Tamari-type wheat-free soy sauce**
	sea salt and freshly ground black pepper

1. Fry the onion in the oil for 3 to 4 minutes.
2. Put the fried onion, mushroom slices, water and soy sauce into a liquidizer, blend and pour into the saucepan.
3. Bring to the boil and simmer for about 5 minutes.
4. Season to taste and serve hot.

sippets

Fry cubes of special wheat-free bread lightly in hot olive oil until golden. Sprinkle into hot soup and serve. Cut the bread into thick slices and then into cubes, before you fry them.

hot vegetable snack

serves one

3 medium	**mushrooms**
1 medium	**tomato**
2 thin slices	**onion**
1 small stick	**celery**
1 tsp	**Tamari-type wheat-free soy sauce**
1 tsp	**white wine or white wine vinegar**
2 tbs	**water**
1 tsp	**freshly chopped parsley**
	sea salt
	freshly ground black pepper

1. Preheat oven to 350°F/180°C/gas mark 4.
2. Slice the mushrooms and tomatoes. Separate the onion into rings and chop the celery finely.
3. In a small casserole, pack the vegetables in layers, ending with a layer of mushrooms. Press down well.
4. In a cup mix the soy sauce, wine or vinegar and water. Pour over the vegetables. Lastly sprinkle with the chopped parsley. Season to taste.
5. Put on the lid and bake for about 30 minutes until the vegetables are tender. Serve hot or cold.

note to cooks   Make sure you press the vegetables down well before cooking or the top layer will be dry.

mushrooms with mint

serves one

1 tbs	sunflower oil
½	garlic clove, peeled
100g/4oz/1 cup	mushrooms
2	fresh tomatoes, peeled and chopped
	fresh mint leaves, chopped
	sea salt
	freshly ground black pepper

1 Heat the oil in a frying pan (skillet).

2 Put in the garlic (crushed), mushrooms, tomatoes and chopped mint.

3 Season and cover with a lid.

4 Simmer for about 12 to 15 minutes.

5 Serve hot with triangles of wheat-free fried bread or sippets.

whitebait

100g/4oz	**whitebait**
	oat flour
3 tbs	**sunflower or soya oil**
	sea salt and freshly ground black pepper
	parsley sprigs
	lemon slice for decoration

1 Wash the fish well under the cold running tap. Drain well in a colander.

2 Put a tablespoonful of oatflour into a paper bag and toss the fish in this until well coated.

3 Heat the oil in a shallow pan and fry the coated fish in this a few at a time. When crisp and brown, drain on kitchen paper and keep hot while you fry the remainder.

4 Serve right away with the parsley and lemon garnish.

note to cooks   To make oat flour, grind porridge oats in a coffee grinder (electric).

tomato starter

A very simple but delicious starter. Use a really good quality tomato – a home-grown one would be ideal.

serves one

1	**tomato**
1 level tsp	**freshly chopped parsley**
1 slice	**onion, chopped very finely**
	sugar
	freshly ground black pepper
	sea salt

1 Cut the tomato into thin slices.
2 Lay overlapping, on a plate, and sprinkle with the parsley and onion plus a few pinches of sugar.
3 Season to taste.
4 Serve cold with wheat-free crispbread and milk-free margarine.

note to cooks   Three chive blades, snipped small with kitchen scissors, can be substituted for the parsley.

liver and mushroom pâté

Not suitable for pregnant women.

¼ kilo/½ lb/8oz	chicken livers
½ medium	onion, peeled and chopped
1 tbs	sunflower oil
1	clove garlic, peeled
¼ kilo/½ lb/8oz	mushrooms, chopped
2–3 tsp	Tamari-type wheat-free soy sauce
¼ tsp	dried thyme
	sea salt
	freshly ground black pepper

1 Cut out all the strings etc., from the livers and discard.

2 Wash and chop livers. Pat dry with kitchen paper.

3 Fry the onion in the oil until soft.

4 Add the chopped livers and crush in the garlic. Turn up the heat and stir with a small wooden spoon or fork. As soon as the livers start to turn brown and crumble, add the mushrooms and soy sauce.

5 Cook while you stir for about 3 or 4 minutes.

6 Leave to cool, then blend, adding the thyme and seasoning to taste.

7 Put into little dishes and store, covered, in the fridge.

note to cooks   Serve with hot wheat-free toast and milk-free margarine for the special dieter and ordinary toast and butter for the rest of the family. A useful starter as it will serve the whole family and can be made well in advance.

crudités

Serve as dips with special mayonnaise as a starter.

Radishes – scrubbed and trimmed.

Celery – scrubbed and trimmed and cut into short lengths.

Carrot – peeled, washed and trimmed and cut into matchstick shapes.

Spring onions (scallions) – washed and trimmed.

Cauliflower – use the crisp white pieces and break into florets after washing well.

Lettuce – use just the heart leaves. Wash and pat dry with a clean tea-towel. Any variety of lettuce will do.

Tomato – only use if you can get small fruits. Wash and leave whole.

Cucumber – leave the skin on and cut into small fingers.

Celeriac – peel and cut into matchsticks.

Fennel – trim and cut into curved matchsticks.

Pepper (Bell pepper) – de-seed and cut into sticks.

note to cooks   A selection of 4 or 5 is ideal, but at least 2 must be brightly coloured.

stuffed mushrooms

Although this makes an unusual starter it can also be a good accompaniment to baked fish or chicken.

serves one

2 to 3	open, largish mushrooms
1 tbs	sunflower oil
½ small	onion, peeled and chopped finely
1 tbs	wheat-free breadcrumbs or cooked rice
1 rasher	back bacon, grilled
2 heaped tsp	chopped fresh parsley
1 heaped tsp	ground almonds
	garlic salt
	freshly ground black pepper
	parsley for garnish

1   Preheat oven to 375°F/190°C/gas mark 5.

2   Wash the mushrooms and remove stalks. Chop just the stalks finely.

3   Heat the oil in a frying pan (skillet) and put in the chopped stalks and onion. Fry over a gentle heat for about 3 to 4 minutes.

4   Sprinkle in the breadcrumbs or cooked rice and fry until brown and crisp.

5   Trim the fat off the grilled bacon and discard. Chop the bacon and add to the fried mixture with the chopped parsley and ground almonds.

6   Season with the garlic salt and pepper to taste.

7   Put the mushroom caps, hollow side up, in a well oiled, shallow, ovenproof dish. Fill the caps with stuffing.

8   Sprinkle with a little oil, cover with a lid and bake for about 25 minutes above centre of oven.

9   Serve hot, garnished with parsley.

note to cooks   If preferred, lean ham (without breadcrumbs) can be used instead of bacon. Just chop and add to stuffing mixture. If you don't have any wheat-free bread to spare try cooked, boiled rice instead.

suggestions for other starters

Other, old favourites that can be served to all the family are melon sprinkled with a little sugar (if not sweet enough), or a mixture of grapefruit and orange slices, or just plain grapefruit.

snacks

As most commercial biscuits and cookies are made with wheat-flour, egg and margarine (which is not milk-free), you will need to make your own at home if you wish to continue eating them for snacks. Store the end results in air-tight containers.

Dried fruit and nuts are useful as snacks. Granola is a cereal-like snack that can be made in bulk to use as required.

granola

This is a useful treat for those who want to put on weight or want their weight to remain steady. It can be eaten warm or cold and makes a good snack at any time of day.

serves one to two

1 heaped tbs	**rolled oats**
1 heaped tbs	**barley flakes**
1 tbs	**sunflower oil**
1 tbs	**chopped mixed nuts, such as almonds, cashews, walnuts and hazelnuts**
1 tbs	**sunflower seeds**
a little	**runny honey, to taste**
1 heaped tbs	**sultanas/golden raisins or raisins, or a mixture**

1 Put the rolled oats, barley flakes and oil in a small, heavy-based pan. Heat gently to allow the flakes to absorb the oil.

2 Add the nuts, seeds and honey and stir over a low heat for about 10 minutes.

3 Turn up the heat to let it brown, then remove from the heat and mix in the dried fruit.

4 Serve like cereal, with soya milk poured over.

note to cooks Barley flakes can be purchased from health-food stores.

savoury nibbles

makes about fifty little crisps

30g/1oz	**porridge oats**
1 tbs	**sunflower oil**
4 tbs	**water**
¼ tsp	**yeast extract**

1   Preheat oven to 450°F/230°C/gas mark 8.

2   Grind the oats to flour in a coffee grinder and put into a bowl.

3   Add the oil and water. Mix well.

4   Put in the yeast extract and beat until you have a thin, smooth batter using a wooden spoon.

5   Grease a baking sheet. Take teaspoons of the batter and drop one third of a teaspoon each time on the baking sheet. The mixture will spread a little to the size of a small coin. Leave space around each one.

6   Bake for about 6 minutes until brown around the edges. Leave to cool on the baking sheet.

7   Serve in a bowl with drinks. Put into a plastic bag or container as part of a lunchbox.

variation   Instead of yeast extract, use 2 good pinches of mild, wheat-free curry powder.

digestive biscuits

makes about twelve

15g/1½oz/1 tbs	barley flour
50g/2oz/5 tbs	ground brown rice
25g/1oz/2½ tbs	sugar
15g/½oz	soya/soy flour (low fat)
3 pinches	powdered cloves
25g/1oz/2½ tbs	special milk-free margarine
	a little water
	extra ground brown rice for rolling out

1   Preheat oven to 325°F/170°C/gas mark 3.
2   Put the first five ingredients into a bowl and mix well.
3   Add the margarine and rub in until the mixture resembles breadcrumbs.
4   Add water, 1 teaspoonful at a time, kneading the mixture until it binds. It should form one ball of dough and leave the bowl clean.
5   Roll out using more ground rice to about 3mm (⅛ inch) thick.
6   Cut into rounds with a pastry cutter and use a spatula to lift them on to a baking sheet.
7   Prick with a fork and bake for about 10 to 12 minutes.
8   Lift off carefully while still warm and leave to cool on a wire rack, when they will go crisp.
9   Store in an air-tight tin.

spiced fruit cookies

50g/2oz/¼ cup	milk-free, wheat-free margarine
100g/4oz/½ cup	ground rice
75g/3oz/1 small	finely grated eating apple
40g/1½oz/2 tbs	sugar
40g/1½oz/¼ cup	dried fruit – currants, sultanas/golden seedless raisins, raisins, chopped pitted prunes, dried apricots, etc.
½ tsp	mixed spice

1 Preheat oven to 450°F/230°C/gas mark 8.

2 Put the margarine and ground rice into a bowl and blend with a fork.

3 Add the remaining ingredients and mix with a wooden spoon until it forms one ball of dough.

4 Oil a baking sheet and drop 10 spoonsful of the mixture on to it.

5 Spread out with a knife into cookie shapes about 6 mm (¼ inch) thick.

6 Bake above centre of oven for 20 to 25 minutes. Allow to cool for a minute and then remove carefully with a spatula and put on to a wire rack to cool.

7 The cookies will crisp as they cool down. When cold, sprinkle with a little more sugar. Eat on the day of baking.

fruit and nuts

A simple snack and one that is easy to carry, combining fruit and nuts. Fruit can be fresh or dried but nuts should be fresh and not processed in any way. Wash dried fruits under the tap and dry on a clean tea-towel.

Try some of these combinations:

a   Dried apricots, raisins and almonds

b   Sultanas (golden seedless raisins), cashews and a fresh banana

c   Apple, raisins and hazelnuts/almonds

d   Dried peaches, almonds and raisins

e   Fresh pear with almonds and cashews

f   Raisins, sultanas (golden seedless raisins), peanuts, almonds and hazelnuts

After preparing, put into a small container with a lid or a small plastic bag. These are very high in calories, so if weight loss is a worry, this type of snack could prove very useful.

You will find most health stores carry a good selection of dried fruits and nuts. Once you have bought a selection you can make up little snacks and store them in small plastic bags in a container so that you may take one out when you want it. This should replace the biscuit tin in your life!

oatcakes

makes twelve

225g/8oz/1½ cups	**medium oatmeal**
2 pinches	**salt**
2 tsp	**sunflower oil**
	fine oatmeal for rolling out

1 Mix the oatmeal and salt together in a bowl, then stir in the oil.

2 Add enough boiling water to make a soft dough. Dust the rolling pin and worktop with fine oatmeal and roll out the dough as thinly as you can.

3 Cut into squares or rectangles with a knife or cut into shapes with cutters.

4 Lightly grease a griddle or heavy-based frying pan (skillet) and cook the oatcakes on both sides until the edges start to curl up.

5 Cool on a wire rack and store in an airtight tin. Spread with honey or jam or serve instead of bread.

main meals

Without wheat, milk and eggs you will not be able to offer omelettes, quiches, pastas, sauces made with milk or anything which contains cheese. Dishes where eggs are used as a binder and where wheat is used for coating are also not on the menu. This means no rissoles, croquettes, fish in batter or breadcrumbs. The main source of carbohydrate will be brown rice and potatoes. Traditional roast lamb or beef (a joint) is permitted but not Yorkshire pudding to go with the beef. Although at first glance it seems as if main meals will have to be rather plain, you will find in this section recipes based on Italian, Indian, French and Chinese food as well as British, adapted for this rather special diet. This should make main mealtimes more interesting.

shepherd's pie

serves three

1 medium	onion, peeled and chopped
1 small	clove garlic, peeled
1 tbs	sunflower oil
1	tomato, chopped
¾ lb/3 cups	minced lamb from precooked joint, trimmed of fat etc. before cooking
1 medium	carrot, grated coarsely
3 tsp	Tamari-type wheat-free soya/soy sauce
3 heaped tsp	cornflour/cornstarch
150ml/½ pint/⅔ cup	water
1 heaped tsp	freshly chopped parsley
3 pinches	dried thyme
1 heaped tsp	tomato purée/paste
3 portions	mashed potato*
	sea salt and freshly ground black pepper

1   Preheat the oven to 375°F/190°C/gas mark 5.

2   Use a saucepan to fry the onion and crushed garlic in the sunflower oil.

3   Add the tomato when the onion begins to brown. Stir while you cook until you have a brown sauce.

4   Put in the minced lamb and grated carrot. Fry gently for about 5 minutes while turning over with a wooden spoon or spatula.

5   Spoon in the Tamari-type wheat-free soya (soy) sauce.

6   Blend the cornflour (cornstarch) and water in a cup. Mix well and add to pan.

7   Sprinkle in the parsley, thyme and tomato purée (paste). Stir well and cook while stirring for another 10 minutes. Season to taste, adding more water if it looks too dry.

8   Transfer to a hot pie dish and cover with the mashed potato. Texture with a fork and make a hole in the centre, right through to the meat, to let out the steam during cooking.

9   Bake on the top shelf for about 20 minutes.

10 Serve hot, golden topped and crisp, with a selection of vegetables (hot).

note to cooks   A tasty way to use up a joint of lamb that won't cut into any more slices. Fresh raw minced lamb can also be used for this recipe but the cooking time for stage 4 will need to be 10 minutes and for stage 7 about 30 to 40 minutes.

* The mashed potato should be made with plain boiled potatoes, milk-free/wheat-free margarine and a little water.

goulash

serves four

	cornflour/cornstarch
4 portions	**braising beef**
3 medium	**onions, peeled**
	sunflower oil
1 medium	**tin/can peeled plum tomatoes**
1–2 level tsp	**paprika (or less) sea salt**

1 Preheat the oven to 300°F/150°C/gas mark 2.

2 Sprinkle a little cornflour (cornstarch) on to a plate.

3 Trim off fat and gristle from meat and discard. Cut trimmed meat into neat cubes.

4 Roll in the cornflour (cornstarch).

5 Cut the onions into quarters and fry in a tablespoonful of oil, using a flameproof casserole.

6 Remove onions while you fry the beef cubes in another tablespoonful of the oil. Turn them over while you fry, to seal the meat.

7 Return onions to the casserole with the meat.

8 Add the tomatoes, paprika* and seasoning. Bring to the boil, put on lid and transfer to the oven for about 2½ hours.

9 Serve with plain boiled rice and a green side salad. Garnish with fried wheat-free bread cut into triangles.

note to cooks   This is a slow-cooked casserole. Fresh tomatoes can be used instead of tinned but they will require peeling. If you find the gravy not rich enough then 2 or 3 teaspoonsful of Tamari-type wheat-free soya (soy) sauce can be added. A good deal of the success of this recipe depends on how tasty the tomatoes are. Some people will appreciate a little less paprika.

*Start with the minimum amount, taste and correct with more if required.

prawns italian

1 medium	onion, peeled and chopped finely
1 tbs	sunflower oil or similar
2	cloves garlic, peeled
50g/2oz/1 cup	mushrooms, sliced
½ medium	green pepper, de-seeded and sliced thinly
4 medium	tomatoes, peeled and chopped
3 tsp	Tamari-type wheat-free soya/soy sauce
¼ kilo/½ lb/8oz	peeled prawns
	sea salt and freshly ground black pepper
2 tbs/2½ tbs	finely chopped fresh parsley

1 Fry the onion in the oil.

2 Crush in the garlic, using a garlic press.

3 Add the mushrooms, green pepper and tomatoes. Bring to the boil and simmer gently for 5 minutes.

4 Add the soya sauce and prawns. Heat through gently and simmer for another 5 minutes. Season to taste.

5 Serve hot, on a bed of plain boiled rice, sprinkled with parsley.

note to cooks   This can be served with a green side salad of lettuce and cucumber, with an oil and vinegar dressing.

fish and chips

1 portion	**cod, plaice or haddock, filleted and washed**
	cornflour/cornstarch
2 tsp	**sunflower or soya oil**
1 portion	**peeled raw potatoes**
	sunflower or olive oil for frying

oven chips:

1 Preheat the oven to 450°F/230°C/gas mark 8.

2 Peel the potatoes and cut them into chips (French fries). Put into a roasting tin (pan) with the oil and turn them over by hand to coat with the oil.

3 Cook on the top shelf of the oven for 20 to 25 minutes or until tender, crisp and golden. Serve hot. If they are ready too soon, put them in the bottom of the oven on a very low heat and they will not spoil. However, they are best when freshly cooked. Serve with peas and grilled tomatoes (if room).

fish:

1 Dip the fish in cornflour (cornstarch) to coat it all over.

2 Heat a little oil in a frying pan (skillet).

3 Fry the fish for about 5 minutes on each side (or less if the fillet is thin) until cooked on the inside and with a crisp golden outside.

4 Drain on kitchen paper and serve hot garnished with lemon.

cold salmon

serves two

1 litre/2 pints/5 cups	**water**
150ml/¼ pint/⅔ cup	**wine vinegar**
1	**onion, sliced**
1	**stick/stalk celery, chopped**
1	**carrot, grated coarsely**
1 heaped tbs	**freshly chopped parsley**
1 tsp	**black peppercorns**
	sea salt to taste
2	**fresh salmon steaks, washed,**
	(cut from the centre of the fish)

1 Put the first seven ingredients into a large saucepan. Boil for about 30 minutes, adding more water if the level goes down too much.

2 Strain and pour back into the pan.

3 Add salt to taste and stir.

4 Put the salmon steaks carefully into the warm stock which should cover the fish. (If it doesn't, add more water.)

5 Bring to the boil and simmer for about 3 minutes.

6 Very carefully, using a large fish slice, turn the steaks without breaking them.

7 Simmer for another 3 minutes and then turn out the heat.

8 Leave the salmon to grow cold in the liquid. It will continue to cook very slowly as it cools down.

9 Lift the fish out very carefully with a fish slice. Drain and put onto plates. Serve cold with salads and boiled new potatoes, sprinkled with freshly chopped parsley and glazed with melted milk-free/wheat-free margarine.

note to cooks   By leaving the salmon in the liquid until required for serving, it will not go dry. Serve for a special occasion – this is still considered to be a luxury fish.

trout

Trout can often be bought more cheaply than cod or haddock. The flesh is pale pink and has a delicate flavour. Buy trout already cleaned. Before cooking, wash and pat dry with kitchen paper. Season before all methods of cooking with sea salt and freshly ground black pepper.

Bake in an oiled, shallow, ovenproof dish that has a lid or cover. Preheat oven to 350°F/180°C/gas mark 4 for about 30 minutes, above centre of oven.

Fry for 5 or 6 minutes each side.

Grill on both sides for 8 to 10 minutes, under a medium grill. Traditional garnish for trout – lemon slices and sprigs of parsley.

trout with almonds

Fry the fish and wipe the pan clean. Keep warm while you fry a sprinkle of flaked almonds in a knob of milk-free margarine. Squeeze fresh lemon juice over the fish and cover with the fried almonds.

baked trout

Put the fish into a well-oiled dish and sprinkle with dried tarragon and 1 to 2 tablespoonsful of white wine. Bake and serve with the juices.

trout with herbs

Coat the fish with cornflour (cornstarch) and fry. Keep hot while you heat a generous knob of milk-free/wheat-free margarine in a small pan. Squeeze in the juice of 1/4 of a lemon and 1/2 a level teaspoonful of mixed herbs. Mix well, pour over the fish and serve.

fish and pepper hotpot

serves two

3 medium	potatoes, peeled and thickly sliced
2	spring onions (scallions), chopped
1 tbs	sunflower oil
1 small	green (bell) pepper, deseeded and cut into strips
½	tin/can peeled plum tomatoes in juice, chopped
1 small	clove garlic, peeled
	salt and freshly ground black pepper
2	cod or haddock fillets, skinned
½	lemon, juice of
1 heaped tsp	finely chopped fresh parsley

1 Preheat the oven to 350°F/180°C/gas mark 4.
2 Boil the potato slices for 15 minutes, then drain and set aside.
3 Fry the spring onions (scallions) in the oil for 1 minute, then add the green (bell) pepper, tomatoes and garlic.
4 Add water to cover, bring to the boil, then reduce the heat and simmer for 15 minutes. Season to taste and spoon into an ovenproof dish.
5 Arrange the fish fillets on top of the pepper mixture and squeeze over the lemon juice. Cover with the potato slices and dot with butter.
6 Bake for 20 minutes, until the fish is cooked. Sprinkle with the parsley and serve with spinach or broccoli.

grilled white fish with herbs

serves one

1 fillet	**white fish (haddock, plaice, cod or turbot)**
1 tsp	**fresh lemon juice**
1 tbs	**freshly chopped parsley**
1 tbs	**freshly chopped chives**
1 tsp	**sunflower oil**
	sea salt
	freshly ground black pepper

1 Wash the fish of your choice.

2 Place on a metal plate or dish and sprinkle with the lemon juice, herbs, oil and seasoning.

3 Leave to marinate in the fridge for about half an hour.

4 Grill for about 4 to 5 minutes each side, under a moderate grill. If the fish starts to look dry, sprinkle with a little more oil.

5 Serve hot with tomatoes (for colour), peas and plain boiled potatoes or rice. Also good with savoury rice.

note to cooks   This recipe can be used for a breakfast dish if the chives are omitted. Serve hot with grilled tomatoes and wheat-free bread spread with milk-free/wheat-free margarine. Fresh salmon fillets or steaks can also be used but omit the chives.

cod portugaise

serves two

3 tbs	fresh lemon juice
3 tbs	sunflower oil
	sea salt
	freshly ground black pepper
1	clove garlic, peeled
1	bayleaf
4	cod fillets or steaks
	Red sauce *(page 90)*
	chopped parsley

1 Make the marinade by mixing the first six ingredients in a dish.
2 Put in the washed raw fish and leave for about 20 minutes. Turn the fish over and leave for another 20 minutes.
3 Preheat oven to 350°F/180°C/gas mark 4.
4 Grease an ovenproof dish with milk-free margarine or sunflower oil. Place the drained fish on this and put on the lid.
5 Bake for about 20 to 30 minutes, depending on thickness of fish.
6 Heat the Red sauce and pour a couple of tablespoonsful over each steak/fillet. Put back in the oven for five minutes.
7 Sprinkle with chopped parsley and serve hot with plain, boiled rice or potatoes and peas.

red sauce

For fish, steak, chops, etc.

2 tbs	**sunflower oil**
1	**clove garlic, peeled**
1 medium	**tin/can tomatoes**
1 heaped tsp	**tomato purée/paste**
few pinches	**dried oregano**
6 sprigs	**fresh parsley, chopped finely**
1 tsp	**sugar**
	freshly ground black pepper
	sea salt

1 Heat the oil in a small pan.

2 Crush in the garlic and lower the heat.

3 Chop the tomatoes and add to the pan.

4 Add the tomato purée (paste), herbs, and sugar. Heat and stir for about 10 minutes.

5 Season to taste. Serve hot.

note to cooks   See recipe for Cod Portugaise (*page 89*) which uses this sauce.

grilled meat

Grilling steak (beef), veal, lamb or pork makes a quick and easy meat course. Steaks, chops or fillets can be rubbed with a cut clove of garlic or sprinkled with herbs for variety. Grill on both sides for a few minutes until tender.

Here are some serving suggestions:

- Grilled steak with fried mushrooms and onions
- Lamb chops rubbed with garlic and sprinkled with rosemary
- Pork chops with stewed apple (as apple sauce)
- Lamb chops sprinkled with dried tarragon and served with grilled tomatoes

See recipe for mint sauce *(page 112)* to serve with plain grilled lamb chops. Stir-fry is also a good vegetable dish to serve with grilled meat.

Good accompaniments are grilled tomatoes, fried mushrooms and onions, green vegetables and potatoes or plain boiled rice.

nut roast

serves two

1	onion, peeled and chopped
1 slice	wheat-free bread, made into crumbs
3 tsp	Tamari-type wheat-free soya/soy sauce
1 heaped tsp	tomato purée/paste
3	tinned/canned tomatoes, chopped
1	grated eating apple
75g/3oz/¾ cup	ground hazelnuts
3 good pinches	dried mixed herbs
	sea salt
	freshly ground black pepper
	oil for greasing

1 Preheat the oven to 425°F/220°C/gas mark 7.

2 Mix the first eight ingredients in a bowl and season.

3 Grease a shallow ovenproof dish. Turn the mixture into this. Flatten with a knife.

4 Bake for about 25 minutes on the top shelf.

5 Serve with green vegetables and either potatoes or plain boiled rice.

nut rissoles

makes five to six

Make the recipe for Nut Roast but instead of turning into a dish, make into flat cakes. Roll in cornflour (cornstarch) to coat and fry in shallow hot oil for about 3 minutes each side. Serve hot.

note to cooks   Nut roasts and rissoles are usually bound with egg to stop them disintegrating. You will find that grated apple does this job just as well. A really tasty and light protein dish. For variety try ground cashews or walnuts, almonds or Brazils, or any mixture. A level tablespoonful of freshly chopped parsley can be used instead of the dried herbs. Serve to the whole family.

gravy

For people who have allergies the complexities of gravy mixes and stock cubes are definitely out. The best approach is to make gravy using the natural juices from grilled or roasted meat, thickened with cornflour (cornstarch) and any vegetable strainings available. To strengthen the stock, a little Tamari-type wheat-free soy sauce can be added. Tamari-type soy sauce is made from soy beans and rice. If you prefer, add a mashed boiled potato for thickening. For more details of the special soy sauce, see page 21.

1 Strain off and discard the fat from meat juices left in the grill pan or roasting tin. It is important to do this well or the gravy will be too greasy.
2 Add the thickening of your choice and rub into the pan with the back of a wooden spoon. This will release any solid juices from the pan/tin as well as distribute the thickening.
3 Heat and cook while you add vegetable strainings or water.
4 Add the Tamari-type wheat-free soya sauce – 2 or 3 teaspoonsful to taste.
5 Bring to the boil and simmer for a couple of minutes. Serve hot.

liver with orange and bacon

Unsuitable for pregnant women.

50g/2oz/1 medium piece	**lamb's liver**
1	**back rasher, lean meat from, chopped**
1 tbs	**vegetable oil**
½	**orange, peeled and sliced**
2 tsp	**Tamari-type wheat-free soya/soy sauce**
1 tbs	**pure orange juice**

1 Cut out any stringy pieces from the liver. Wash, dry and cut into small pieces.

2 Heat the oil in a frying pan (skillet) and put in the liver and bacon. Fry gently while turning to cook evenly for 5 minutes.

3 Put in the orange slices, soya (soy) sauce and orange juice. Heat through gently.

4 Serve hot with green vegetables and either plain boiled brown rice or potatoes.

variation   If you prefer a thicker gravy, dip the liver pieces in cornflour (cornstarch) before frying. (Seasoning is added at the table.)

kebabs

This is a quick way of cooking food for a special dieter when the rest of the family is having quite a different meal. It is also an easy dish to take with you if going to someone else's home for a meal. All the hostess has to do is grill it for you, saving both of you worry and trouble.

Basically, kebabs are small portions of fish, meat and vegetables grilled on a long skewer. Variations are endless and they look most attractive. When grilled they can be served on a bed of plain boiled brown rice.

Before grilling, brush the meat or fish with sunflower oil.

pork kebabs

50g/2oz/ 1 medium-sized piece	**trimmed pork fillet**
4	**cubes of pineapple or pieces of apple**
¼	**green pepper, deseeded and quartered**
1 medium	**tomato, quartered**
2 medium	**button mushrooms**
	olive oil
	sea salt and freshly ground black pepper

1 Cut the meat into about 4 or 5 pieces.
2 Assemble on 2 skewers, putting the pineapple next to the meat and the various vegetables etc. in between.
3 Brush with oil, season and grill under a medium heat for 8 to 10 minutes or until cooked through, turning to ensure even cooking.

lamb kebabs

50g/2oz/	trimmed lamb from a chump chop,
1 medium-sized piece	cut into 4 pieces
2 small	tomatoes, cut in half
2	button mushrooms, cut in half
4	fresh mint leaves
¼	red pepper, deseeded and quartered
	olive oil

1 Assemble on 2 skewers, putting the mint leaves next to the meat, and the vegetables in between.

2 Brush with oil, season and grill, turning to ensure even cooking.

other items to use are:

- Stoned prunes, soaked overnight
- Dried apricot halves, soaked for 3 or 4 hours
- Cubes of lamb's liver
- Pieces of prepared kidney
- Cubes of grilling steak, trimmed of fat
- Cubes of cod fillet and thick slices of lemon

savoury rice

1 medium	onion, peeled and chopped
1 tbs	sunflower oil or similar
1	mushroom, chopped
½	red pepper, deseeded and chopped
1	carrot, scrubbed and chopped
1	stick/stalk celery, washed and chopped
2	tender cabbage or spinach leaves, shredded after trimming
1 portion	cooked brown rice
	sea salt and freshly ground black pepper to taste

1 Fry the onion gently in the oil for a few minutes.
2 Add the prepared vegetables and a little water to prevent sticking.
3 Cook with the lid on tightly for about 6 or 7 minutes.
4 Add the cooked rice and mix everything together. Cook until the rice has heated through.
5 Season and add the lemon juice, if liked.
6 Serve hot with fish or meat.

variation   Other kinds of vegetables can be used according to season – green beans, peas, turnips, parsnips, broad beans (Windsor beans) etc. If you want to use tomato this is best served as a garnish as it is very soft when cooked and tends to make the dish too moist. If serving with fish, sprinkle with a little fresh lemon juice. If serving with meat, sprinkle with a little chopped (fresh) parsley.

prawn savoury

Make Savoury Rice and add 1 heaped tablespoonful of peeled prawns for each person. Garnish with lemon.

savoury rice with bacon

Make Savoury Rice. For each person grill one rasher of back bacon. Remove and discard fat and chop remainder into small pieces. Add to the savoury rice and serve hot.

chicken and herb casserole

This is an easy meal for one person and useful if the rest of the family is to eat something different.

½ medium	**onion, peeled and sliced**
2 tsp	**vegetable oil**
2	**mushrooms, sliced**
1	**carrot, scrubbed and sliced**
1 small	**tin/can tomatoes**
2 tsp	**Tamari-type wheat-free soya/soy sauce**
1	**boned chicken breast**
1 large	**potato, peeled and sliced thinly**
2 pinches or	**dried rosemary**
3 pinches	**dried tarragon**
	sea salt and freshly ground black pepper

1 Preheat the oven to 400°F/200°C/gas mark 6.

2 Fry the onion in the oil until transparent.

3 Add the mushrooms, carrot, tomatoes and soya (soy) sauce.

4 Transfer to a warmed casserole. Stir and lay the chicken breast in the centre.

5 Cover with layers of the potato.

6 Season with salt and pepper and sprinkle with the chosen herb.

7 Put the lid on and bake for about an hour.

8 Spoon on to a warmed plate and serve.

note to cooks   Serve this casserole with a green vegetable such as spinach, beans, fresh peas, sprouts or cabbage, lightly cooked. Alternatively, offer a green salad as a side dish. Follow with a fruit salad for an easy but well-balanced meal.

chicken curry

This is a good meal to take with you when you have been invited to dinner in someone else's home, saving the hosts the worry of cooking two separate meals. Either get them to provide you with plain boiled rice or take your own. To make a richer stock add tomato juice instead of water.

serves one

½ medium	onion, peeled and sliced
2 tsp	vegetable oil
1	mushroom, sliced
2	tomatoes, chopped
2 tsp	Tamari-type wheat-free soya/soy sauce
1	boned chicken breast or 2 legs (unboned)
1 heaped tsp	wheat-free curry powder
	sea salt
sprinkling	sultanas/golden seedless raisins or raisins
½	eating apple, cored and sliced
	water
1 heaped tsp	cornflour/cornstarch

1 Cook the onion in the oil in a flameproof casserole, frying for about 4 minutes.

2 Add the mushrooms, tomatoes and soya (soy) sauce.

3 Put in the chicken and cook for about 2 minutes on each side to seal.

4 Sprinkle in the curry powder, salt to taste, the dried fruit and the apple slices.

5 Pour in enough water to cover and bring to the boil. Simmer gently with the lid on for about 45 minutes.

6 Mix the cornflour (cornstarch) with a little water and pour into the casserole. Stir until it thickens.

7 Serve on a bed of hot brown rice, plain boiled.

lemon chicken

This is a spicy Chinese dish. Serve hot with plain, boiled brown rice.

serves two to three

1 tbs	sherry
2	spring onions/scallions
1 small piece	root ginger
3 portions	cooked chicken, boned and trimmed
1 tbs	sunflower or soya/soy oil
1	stick/stalk celery
2 medium	mushrooms
½ medium	green pepper
1 tbs	Tamari-type wheat-free soya/soy sauce (thin)
1	lemon, rind of

1 Put the sherry into a basin.
2 Chop the spring onions (scallions), peel and shred the ginger and add to the sherry.
3 Mix in the chicken, cut into small pieces. Leave for about 20 minutes so that the chicken will absorb the flavour of the sherry etc.
4 Put the oil in a deep frying pan (skillet).
5 Chop the celery, slice the mushrooms and green pepper. Fry in the oil while you stir for about 2 minutes.
6 Add the chicken mixture and continue cooking for 2 minutes.
7 Stir in the soya (soy) sauce and lemon rind (coarsely grated).

chinese fried rice

serves two

1 generous tbs	**sunflower or soya/soy oil**
2	**spring onions/scallions, chopped**
3 or 4	**mushrooms, sliced**
1 slice	**cooked ham (without breadcrumb coating), trimmed of fat and diced**
2 heaped tbs	**cooked, peeled prawns**
150g/6oz/1 cup	**cooked long-grain rice**
2 tsp	**Tamari-type wheat-free soya/soy sauce**
2 heaped tbs	**cooked, diced vegetables**

1 Heat the oil in a deep frying pan (skillet).

2 Put in the onions and mushrooms and fry while you stir for 3 or 4 minutes.

3 Add all remaining ingredients and stir-fry for another 4 or 5 minutes.

4 Serve hot.

sweet and sour fish

serves two

1 heaped tbs	cornflour/cornstarch
2 portions	cod fillets, cut into cubes
	vegetable oil for frying
1	onion, peeled and sliced
4	mushrooms, sliced
3 tbs	tomato juice
1 tbs	wine vinegar
2 tsp	sugar
2 tbs	water
1 tbs	cornflour/cornstarch for sauce

1   Put the heaped tablespoonful cornflour (cornstarch) into a paper bag and put in a few of the fish cubes. Close the bag and shake well to coat fish all over. Continue until all the cubes are coated.

2   Heat some oil – about a tablespoonful will do – in a small saucepan and put in the onion. Fry for 3 or 4 minutes. Put in the mushrooms and fry for another 3 minutes. Transfer to a dish and keep hot while you fry the fish.

3   Fry the coated fish cubes in hot oil until golden brown. Add to the onion/mushrooms and keep warm, in a bowl or dish.

4   In a small saucepan, mix the tomato juice, vinegar, sugar, water and cornflour (cornstarch) to make the sauce. Stir well and heat to boiling point. Simmer, while stirring, to make a thick sauce. Taste to see if it is sweet enough. If not, add a little more of the sugar.

5   Serve immediately with plain boiled rice and stir-fry vegetables. The sauce should be poured over the fish/mushrooms.

beef casserole with orange

Use a flameproof casserole.

serves two to three

1 heaped tbs	cornflour/cornstarch
	sea salt and freshly ground black pepper
350g/¾ lb/12 oz	braising beef, trimmed and cut into small cubes
1 medium	onion, peeled and sliced
½	green pepper, deseeded and chopped
1 tbs	vegetable oil
1	orange, grated rind and juice of
1 tbs	Tamari-type wheat-free soya/soy sauce
	water
1 tbs	chopped fresh parsley to garnish

1 Put the cornflour (cornstarch) into a paper bag. Season with salt and pepper, then add the meat cubes and toss to coat.

2 Fry the onion and pepper in the oil until soft.

3 Add the meat and fry while turning to seal, until evenly browned.

4 Transfer to a casserole with a lid. Stir in the orange rind, juice and soya (soy) sauce.

5 Top up with water, bring to the boil and put on the lid.

6 Bake in a preheated oven at 325°F/170°C/gas mark 3 for about 1½ hours.

7 Serve hot, sprinkled with parsley and accompanied by baked jacket potatoes and green vegetables.

onion and potato bake

serves four

4 large	**potatoes, peeled**
4 medium	**onions**
50g/2oz/¼ cup	**milk-free margarine**
1 heaped tsp	**freshly chopped parsley**

1 Cut each potato into 4 pieces and boil in salted water for about 15 minutes.
2 Strain and cool a little. Slice thickly.
3 Preheat oven to 400°F/200°C/gas mark 6.
4 Peel the onions and chop or slice thinly.
5 Melt the margarine in a frying pan (skillet) and fry the onion for about 3 or 4 minutes.
6 Put the potato slices into a hot dish and spread the onion mixture over the top.
7 Finish cooking in the oven on the top shelf for about another 30 minutes.
8 Serve straight from the oven, sprinkled with the parsley.

note to cooks   This dish has a rather sweet taste on account of the slow cooking of the onions. Most people prefer it without seasoning. Good with salad and lean cold meat such as chicken or ham (without breadcrumb coating).

pork chops with apple salad

serves two

2	lean pork chops
1	eating apple, grated (leave the skin on)
1 heaped tsp	sultanas/golden seedless raisins
1	stick/stalk celery, chopped
6	lettuce leaves, torn into pieces
2	tomatoes, sliced
	squeeze of fresh lemon juice
	sprinkling of sugar
	sea salt and freshly ground black pepper

1   Grill the pork chops on a metal grid – about 10 minutes each side.
2   Combine the apple, sultanas (golden seedless raisins), celery, lettuce and tomatoes in a bowl.
3   Sprinkle over the lemon juice and sugar. Season to taste.
4   Serve the chops on hot plates and the salad on side plates.

note to cooks   Young, tender spinach leaves can be used instead of lettuce leaves.

chicken and mushroom risotto

This is a useful dish to take with you when going out to eat in someone else's house. It looks very appetizing and can be eaten hot or cold.

serves one

1 small	**onion, chopped**
1 tsp	**sunflower or soya/soy oil**
2	**mushrooms, sliced**
1 portion	**cooked chicken, cut into small pieces**
	water
1 tsp	**Tamari-type wheat-free soya/soy sauce**
150g/6oz/1 cup	**cooked long-grain brown rice**
	sea salt and freshly ground black pepper

1 Fry the onion in the oil until transparent.
2 Put in the mushrooms and chicken, adding a little water to prevent sticking. Stir-fry for 3 or 4 minutes.
3 Add the soya (soy) sauce and the rice and stir well. Continue cooking while you stir for another 3 or 4 minutes.
4 Season to taste and serve hot accompanied by a green salad.

roast lamb

leg of lamb (lean)

1 tbs   **sunflower oil**

1   Weigh the joint to find out how long it should be cooked for. Allow 20 minutes per half kilo (to the pound) and 20 minutes over.

2   Preheat oven at 425°F/220°C/gas mark 7.

3   Put the joint into a roasting tin, spoon over the oil, put in the centre of the oven and cook for the amount of time you have calculated.

note to cooks   Roast potatoes can be cooked at the same time on the top shelf. Serve with green vegetables in season and mint sauce. The gravy can be made from the meat juices left in the pan after straining off the fat. Serve cold with mashed potato and salad.

roast lamb with garlic and rosemary

Roast a leg of lamb as above but prepare for the oven by pricking the joint all over with a fork. Crush 2 or 3 cloves of garlic and spread the paste all over the meat. Sprinkle with fresh or dried rosemary leaves. Serve hot or cold.

mint sauce:

2 heaped tbs	**freshly chopped mint leaves**
3 tsp	**sugar**
2 tsp	**boiling water**
2 tbs	**wine vinegar**

1 Put the chopped mint into a jug.
2 Add the sugar and mix well.
3 Add the boiling water which will help to dissolve the sugar.
4 Stir in the vinegar.
5 Serve with hot plain roast lamb, peas, carrots and roast potatoes.

roast beef

Cook as for roast lamb but allow 15 minutes per half kilo (pound) and 15 minutes over. If the joint is very lean you may need to spoon over a tablespoonful of sunflower or soya (soy) oil before cooking. This will give the traditional 'underdone' pink and red meat. If you prefer it well cooked, use the same instructions as for roast lamb. Serve with greens, roast potatoes and carrots or parsnips.

.

good, old-fashioned stew

This is a useful basic recipe because the whole course is cooked in one container. The vegetables can be varied according to what is in season or available – peas, broad beans, celery, green beans, turnips, parsnips, etc. An ideal meal to save washing up and effort in the kitchen! It can be served to the whole family and any leftovers can be reheated the following day. A little wheat-free curry powder will make it into a curry to be eaten with plain boiled rice.

In terms of nutritional value this recipe is worth a closer look. The proportions of fat to protein to fibre are excellent, providing the meat is trimmed of all visible fat before cooking. Fats are both saturated and unsaturated. None of the vegetables need to be strained so all juices are eaten. It is not oversalted. Vegetables form the basis of the dish and if these are all fresh so much the better. If served with a dark green vegetable such as kale, broccoli or cabbage this dish is really good. It is the kind of food that our great-grandparents would have enjoyed – a simple, well-balanced meal, easy to prepare, nourishing and appetizing.

serves four to five

4 portions	**braising steak**
	cornflour/cornstarch
4	**onions, peeled and sliced**
	sunflower oil
¼ kilo/½ lb	**carrots, peeled and sliced**
4 or 5	**mushrooms, sliced**
1 tbs	**Tamari-type wheat-free soya/soy sauce**
	sea salt
	freshly ground black pepper
1 medium	**red or green pepper, deseeded and sliced**
4 large	**potatoes (or equivalent), peeled if old and quartered**
2 heaped tbs	**cooked beans – haricot, navy etc. (optional)**
	extra vegetables in season

1 Trim the meat of fat and gristle. Cut into cubes and roll in cornflour (cornstarch).

2 Fry the onion in a tablespoonful of sunflower oil, until it begins to brown, using a large saucepan or flameproof casserole.

3 Put in the meat cubes and another spoonful of oil. Fry while turning over for 3 to 4 minutes to seal the meat.

4 Add the soya (soy) sauce, all the vegetables (including the extras), the beans if you are using them and enough water to cover.

5 Season. Bring to the boil while you stir. Transfer to a casserole if necessary and put into an oven preheated to 425°F/220°C/gas mark 7, middle shelf. Cook for about 1 to 1¼ hours.

6 Serve hot with chunks of wheat-free bread for the special dieter and ordinary bread for the rest of the family.

note to cooks   If the level of the liquid in the casserole goes too low, top up with boiling water. Usually the potatoes will help to thicken the rich gravy, but if you are using new ones that remain firm you may need something more, e.g. put 1 to 2 teaspoons of cornflour (cornstarch) into a cup with 3 tablespoonsful water. Mix to a smooth cream. Stir into the casserole. Cover again and put back into the oven.

bolognese sauce

serves four to five

1 tbs	sunflower oil
2 medium	onions, peeled and sliced finely
2 rashers	back bacon, trimmed of fat
50g/2oz/½ cup	chicken livers
¼ kilo/½ lb/8oz	minced beef (raw)
2	cloves garlic, peeled
2 level tsp	cornflour/cornstarch
¾ litre/1½ pints/3¾ cups	water
¼ kilo/½ lb/8oz	diced mixed vegetables
1 medium	tin/can tomatoes, chopped
1 tbs	tomato purée/paste
1 tbs	Tamari-type wheat-free soy sauce
	a bouquet garni

1 Heat the oil in a large pan. Fry the onions while stirring, until soft.

2 Cut the bacon into small squares. Cut out and discard the stringy parts of the livers and chop.

3 Add to the onion and fry gently while you stir for another couple of minutes.

4 Put in the minced beef and turn up the heat to fry briskly for about 3 minutes, turning the mixture over to brown the meats.

5 Peel the garlic. Crush into the meat mixture.

6 Mix the cornflour (cornstarch) in a cup with a little of the water. Add to the pan and stir.

7 Put in the vegetables, chopped tomatoes, tomato purée (paste) and soya (soy) sauce.

8 Pour in the remainder of the water and bring to the boil while stirring.

9 Season and add the bouquet garni.

10 Simmer for about 30 minutes, giving the occasional stir.

11 Take out the bouquet garni and serve hot with plain, boiled rice and a green side salad.

note to cooks   The rich dark sauce complements the rice. Serve with mixed green side salad and follow with fruit for a balanced meal.

If the vegetables are fresh, this sauce can be cooked, allowed to cool and then frozen for future use in individual portions.

liver provençale

Not suitable for pregnant women.

serves one

100g/4oz/2 small pieces	lamb's liver
	cornflour/cornstarch
	sea salt and freshly ground black pepper
2 tsp	sunflower or soya/soy oil
1 heaped tsp	milk-free margarine
3 or 4 sprigs	fresh parsley, finely chopped
1 small	clove garlic, crushed
1 tsp	wine vinegar

1 Trim the liver of all strings etc., and cut into thin slices.
2 Sprinkle with a little cornflour (cornstarch), salt and pepper.
3 Heat the oil in a small, heavy-based frying pan (skillet) and put in the slices of liver. Cook for about 1 minute each side.
4 Put on to a hot plate and keep warm.
5 Melt the knob of margarine in the frying pan (skillet) but do not let it brown.
6 Add the parsley and garlic and stir.
7 Add the vinegar, which will make it sizzle.
8 Pour over the liver and serve with mashed potatoes and hot vegetables or a green salad.

vegetables for main meals

mashed potatoes

boiled (floury) potatoes

milk-free, wheat-free margarine or olive oil

hot water

sea salt and freshly ground black pepper

ground nutmeg

1 Mash the potatoes while still hot.
2 Add a knob of margarine or a teaspoonful of olive oil for each portion and let it melt into the potato.
3 Beat in enough hot water to make the potatoes creamy.
4 Season to taste and add a small pinch of nutmeg for each portion.
5 Serve hot with a suitable meat or fish dish and vegetables.

jacket potatoes

Choose old potatoes and scrub with a hard brush to remove any dirt. Cut out any 'eyes' or discoloured parts with a sharp knife. Pierce the skin with the point of the knife in several places. (This is to let out steam during baking.) Put a metal skewer through the centre of each one and place on a baking sheet. Bake in a preheated oven at 425°F/220°C/gas mark 7 for about an hour or until the flesh is soft. Eat the whole potato including the skin and serve with milk-free margarine.

crispy roast potatoes

Use old potatoes for best results.

potatoes, peeled and cut into evenly sized pieces

olive oil

1 Preheat the oven to 425°F/220°C/gas mark 7.
2 Put the potatoes into a roasting tin (pan) and spoon in 1 teaspoon of oil for each medium potato. Turn over the potato pieces by hand until they are coated with the oil.
3 Cook on the top shelf of the oven for about 45 to 50 minutes, until the potatoes are crisp and golden. Serve hot.

note to cooks If the potatoes are ready too soon, leave them in the bottom of the oven until you are ready to serve. (Not applicable to fan ovens.)

spinach

¼ kilo/½ lb/8oz   **fresh raw spinach per person**

sea salt

water

1   Fill the sink with cold water and wash spinach really well.
2   Tear off the green parts of the larger leaves and discard stalks.
3   Put into a large saucepan with a sprinkling of salt and 1 tablespoonful of water.
4   Put the lid on and cook gently for 10 to 15 minutes until tender. Poke the leaves down with a wooden spoon after the first 5 minutes.
5   Drain well in a colander. Chop with a sharp knife and serve hot.

note to cooks   Spinach contains a good deal of moisture and does not need to be cooked in water. The natural juices will run out of the leaves during cooking. The strainings can be used for enriching soup, gravy, etc.

root vegetables

turnips, carrots, swede (rutabaga) and parsnips
prepare by trimming and scrubbing,
then cut into pieces and cook as follows:

1   Put into a saucepan which has enough boiling, salted water to come halfway up the vegetables.
2   Bring to the boil and simmer with the lid on until tender but not soft.
3   Strain and serve hot.

note to cooks   Young vegetables will take only 20 to 25 minutes. Older vegetables may take a little longer. Parsnips can be roasted in the oven as for roast potatoes.

greens

Prepare by trimming off all discoloured leaves etc. On outside leaves, tear the leaf away from tough stalks and discard the latter. Sprouts should be trimmed at the base and cut into four.

After preparation and thorough washing, cook sprouts, cabbage, spring greens, sprout tops, kale and broccoli in the same way.

1   Put 5mm (1/4 inch) water into a saucepan and bring to the boil.
2   Add a sprinkling of sea salt and put in the prepared greens, poking them down (leafy ones) with a wooden spoon.
3   Put the lid on and cook gently after bringing to the boil. Seven to 10 minutes should be ample.
4   Serve immediately.

note to cooks   Many cooks start with good quality fresh greens and then ruin them by boiling in large quantities of water and by adding bicarbonate of soda (baking soda). Most of the goodness escapes into the water which is then thrown away, and the bicarbonate of soda (baking soda) finishes off most of the vitamins! (It is very important to eat at least one large portion of greens per day. They should be fresh and not frozen or tinned for maximum nutrition.)

broad beans (windsor beans)

Shell and cook as for root vegetables.

cauliflower

Trim off tough outer leaves. Cut a slice off the root part at the base and discard. Wash thoroughly and cut into 6 or 8 sections, depending on size. Cook as for greens.

peas

Shell and cook as for greens.

green beans

Cut off strings (if necessary). Cut into short lengths. Cook as for greens.

stir-fry vegetables

All vegetables can be cooked by the stir-fry method, which is not only quick but retains the maximum of vitamins and minerals possible for cooked vegetables.

1 Prepare a selection of vegetables including onion.
2 Cut into thin slices or shred, whichever is suitable.
3 Put a tablespoonful of sunflower or soya oil into a wok or deep frying pan (skillet) and heat.
4 Put in the onion and fry for a minute.
5 Gradually put in the vegetables, the hardest ones first (carrots, potatoes, turnips, etc.) and the softest last (cucumber, beansprouts, etc.). Stir-fry, turning the vegetables over gently and moving them to the outside of the pan as they become softened.
6 If the vegetables begin to stick, then add a little water.

note to cooks   The juices of all the vegetables will accumulate at the bottom of the pan. If you add 2 or 3 teaspoonsful of Tamari-type wheat-free soy sauce you will have a delicious gravy. (This way of cooking vegetables does not usually need seasoning.)

cold meat and salads

Beef, lamb and pork slices cut off a cold joint roasted the day before make an easy meal with salad and jacket potatoes. Here are some salad suggestions and instructions for the jacket potatoes.

seasonal salads

A healthy diet should contain a good portion of raw salad every day. This can be eaten with cold meat, fish or nuts and hot potatoes baked in their jackets, plain boiled or mashed.

Some cooked vegetables such as broad beans (Windsor beans), green beans and peas can be used to make a salad interesting. Brightly coloured vegetables such as carrot, tomatoes, red pepper and beetroot (beet) can also be used to add colour to the more dull-looking vegetables like swede (rutabaga), parsnip and white cabbage, etc.

Here are two lists of salad vegetables and fruit. Two items from each list, combined and dressed with either a lemon dressing or an oil and vinegar dressing, a sprinkling of sea salt, freshly ground black pepper and a little sugar (optional) will make interesting salads for one.

soft/moist

Cucumber, 25mm (1 inch) sliced or chopped

Spring onion (scallion), chopped small

Cooked green beans, 2 heaped tablespoonsful

Cooked broad beans (Windsor beans), 1 heaped tablespoonful

Peas, cooked, 2 heaped tablespoonsful

Raw mushrooms, 2 medium-sized, chopped or sliced

Eating apple, ½ a medium fruit, grated or sliced, skin left on

Grapes, 6 to 8 de-pipped

¼ peeled orange, sliced

½ tangerine, satsuma or clementine, divided into segments

Sultanas (golden seedless raisins) or raisins, 1 tablespoonful

Cold cooked haricot (dried) or butter (Lima) beans, 1 heaped tablespoonful

1 tomato, sliced

crisp/crunchy

Carrot, 1 small grated

Raw peas, 1 heaped tablespoonful

Parsnip, ½ medium-sized, grated coarsely

Swede (rutabaga) or beetroot (beet), 25mm (1 inch) cubes or grated

¼ green, red or yellow pepper, chopped

Watercress, ¼ of a bunch of sprigs

Lettuce, 4 leaves

Cress, ½ packet

Spinach or curly kale, 3 young leaves, shredded

Brussels sprouts, 4 shredded

Cabbage, 1 portion of red, green or white, shredded finely

Cauliflower, 4 florets

Beansprouts, 2 heaped tablespoonsful, chopped or left whole

Celery, 1 stick (stalk), chopped or sliced

rice salad

serves one

2 heaped tbs	**cooked brown rice**
1	**spring onion (scallion)**
1 heaped tbs	**chopped red (bell) pepper**
sprinkle	**sultanas (golden seedless raisins)**
1 tbs	**cold cooked peas**
2 or 3	**walnuts/English walnuts, chopped**
1 small	**mushroom, chopped**
1 tbs	**sunflower oil**
2 tsp	**lemon juice**
	sea salt
	freshly ground black pepper
	sugar

1 Put the first seven ingredients into a small bowl.

2 Mix well.

3 Put the sunflower oil and lemon juice into a cup and mix with a teaspoon.

4 Season with the salt and pepper and enough sugar to make a slightly sweet dressing.

5 Dress the salad and serve immediately with cold meat or fish.

note to cooks   If you wish to garnish the salad use a slice of lemon and a sprig of parsley.

lemon dressing

1 tbs	**fresh lemon juice**
3 tbs	**sunflower or soya/soy oil**
1 tsp	**sugar**
	sea salt and freshly ground black pepper to taste

1   Put all ingredients into a screw-top jar.

2   Shake vigorously to combine before sprinkling over salads.

note to cooks   This dressing has a very fresh taste. It is especially good for salads which contain apple, raw mushrooms and cooked peas as the lemon will stop them turning brown or yellow.

sesame oil dressing

Put 1 tablespoon of wine vinegar, 2 tablespoons of sunflower oil and 1 tablespoon of sesame oil into a screwtop jar. Add 1 teaspoon of caster sugar and 2 pinches of salt. Shake well before using.

This dressing will perk up most kinds of salads.

raspberry vinegar dressing

Put 2 teaspoonsful of wine vinegar and 2 teaspoonsful raspberry vinegar into a screwtop jar with 2 tablespoonsful of sunflower oil and 1 teaspoonful of caster sugar. Shake well before using.

Good on salads with cabbage and root vegetables or green salads.

oil and vinegar dressing

Put 1 tablespoonful of wine or cider vinegar and 3 tablespoonsful of sunflower oil into a screw-top jar. Shake well before using. (This dressing should be used to moisten salads, not to swamp them.) Extra virgin oil can be used instead of sunflower oil if preferred.

minty dressing

1 tsp	**freshly chopped mint leaves**
1 tsp	**French mustard (wheat-free)**
2 tsp	**lemon juice**
2 tsp	**finely chopped onion or chives**
	sugar or fructose

1 Put the first four ingredients into a screw-top jar and put the top on. Shake vigorously to combine.

2 Taste and add sugar or fructose to taste. Shake again.

note to cooks   Use leftover cold, boiled new potatoes and peas. Serve with cold roast lamb and salad.

french dressing

makes about 150ml/¼ pint

2 tbs	white wine vinegar
6 tbs	sunflower oil
1 tsp	French Mustard (wheat-free)
½	clove garlic, peeled and crushed
1 tsp	sugar or fructose
	sea salt and freshly ground black pepper

1 Put the first five ingredients into a screw-top jar.
2 Add seasoning to taste.
3 Put on the top and shake well until all ingredients have combined.
4 Store in the fridge and use as required. Always shake well before using.

savoury rice

This is a useful dish as it adds variety and colour to plain grilled meat or fish without having to use several saucepans.

1 Prepare a selection of vegetables, including spring onions (scallions), cut into small dice or shred. Allow 2 heaped tablespoons mixed vegetables per portion.

2 Put a tablespoon of sunflower oil into a small saucepan. Heat and fry the onion for a minute, without letting it brown.

3 Add the prepared vegetables and add a little water, enogh to cover. Put on the lid and cook over a medium heat for a few minutes until vegetables are tender but still crisp and the liquid reduced.

4 Stir in 2 to 3 heaped tablespoons of cooked rice per person. Heat through, season with salt and freshly ground black pepper.

note to cooks   Suitable vegetables for this dish are: mushrooms, red and green (bell) peppers, green beans, peas, carrots, courgettes, brussels sprouts, leeks, turnip, parsnip, celeriac, celery. A combination of three or four from this list plus spring onions will be sufficient.

puddings

The items you will miss on this special kind of diet are mainly the ones made with cow's milk and eggs. You may not serve ordinary milk puddings or quick whipped desserts, ice cream or yogurt and so will have to rely rather heavily on fruit puddings. In its simplest form this type of pudding is really no trouble at all, cheap and high in vitamins. The seasons bring us a good variety of fruit and imports of more exotic kinds of fruit add even more interest and variety.

Use fresh fruit, not tinned or frozen, for maximum nutrition and flavour. The following may sound rather simple in the way of recipes but they are all delicious and easy to prepare. Remember, you may not have cream or custard so use only the best quality fruit.

fruit salad

Fruit salad is always refreshing. Peel and slice fruits so that they are easy to eat. Sweeten to taste with a little sugar or honey and moisten with fresh orange juice. Try the following combinations for variety.

1 small	**eating pear**
3 or 4	**peeled, de-stoned and sliced lychees**
8	**melon cubes**

Good to follow a Chinese main course.

1 small	**eating apple**
4 or 5	**strawberries**
a few	**melon cubes or banana slices**

½	**kiwi fruit, peeled and sliced**
½	**orange, sliced**

5 or 6	**seedless grapes**
1	**fresh peach, peeled, stoned and sliced**
handful	**raspberries or stoned, sweet cherries**

orange and grapefruit slices mixed

Some fruits are nicest eaten on their own, such as figs and nectarines, but the fruit must be really good or it will be a disappointment. Serve strawberries or raspberries with a little sugar. Merely wash the fruit and remove the hulls. Serve in a glass dish. There are many varieties of apples and pears in the shops, as well as plums, grapes and soft fruits such as peaches and apricots.

stewed fruit

The more sour types of fruit can be stewed and sweetened with sugar or honey: apples, cooking pears, plums, apricots, gooseberries, black and redcurrants, peaches, damsons and greengages.

1 Prepare the fruit – either a single type of fruit or a mixture.
2 Cut into pieces or slices and put into a saucepan with a little water and sugar to taste.
3 Bring slowly to the boil and then simmer until tender.
4 Serve hot or cold.

Some fruit contains more moisture than others. Rhubarb can be stewed without any water at all, provided you stir while it cooks. Apples and plums need very little water.

Good mixtures are:

- **Apple and rhubarb**
- **Apple and blackcurrant**
- **Peach and redcurrant**
- **Plum and pear**
- **Peach and raspberry**
- **Apricot and raspberry**

At the end of the soft fruit season and when prices are low because of a glut or an extra good crop, try a *compote* of apple, pear, plum, blackcurrant, redcurrant, damson, etc., as available.

apple dessert

1 medium	cooking apple, peeled, cored and sliced
	brown sugar to taste
2 tsp	sunflower oil
1 tbs	medium oatmeal
2 tsp	runny honey

1 Put the apple in a small pan with 1 tablespoon of water and cook gently until tender.
2 Beat to a purée with a wooden spoon. Sweeten to taste and put into a glass dish to cool.
3 Heat the oil in a small pan and fry the oatmeal for 3 minutes, stirring constantly, until lightly toasted. Stir in the honey, then remove from the heat and leave to cool.
4 Put the apple into a glass serving dish. Sprinkle the oatmeal topping over the apple purée and chill before serving.

apricot tart with nuts

A refreshing pudding that can be served all year round, hot or cold.

filling:

150g/6oz/1 cup	**dried apricots**
2 heaped tsp	**sugar**
¼ litre/½ pint/1⅓ cups	**cold water**
2 tsp	**fresh lemon juice**
25g/1oz/¼ cup	**chopped, shelled nuts**

pastry:

50g/2oz/¼ cup	**milk-free margarine**
100g/4oz/½ cup	**ground brown rice**
75g/3oz/1 small	**grated eating apple**

1 Preheat oven to 425°F/220°C/gas mark 7.
2 Pick over and wash apricots before chopping into small pieces.
3 Put into a saucepan with the sugar, water and lemon juice. Bring to the boil and simmer until all the water has been absorbed.
4 Use a fork to blend the margarine, ground rice and apple. Knead until one ball of dough is formed. Grease an enamel pie-plate and put the dough in the centre. Flatten with the palm and fingers until it has spread evenly over the plate. Raise a slight edge all the way round with the fingers.
5 Spread the filling evenly over the pastry and sprinkle with the nuts.
6 Bake for 20 to 25 minutes on the top shelf and serve hot or cold in slices.

variation   If preferred, sprinkle with a mixture of sunflower seeds and sesame seeds instead of the nuts. A sprinkle of powdered cinnamon in the pastry will make this tart spicy.

grape jelly

A light and delicately flavoured dessert.

serves three

500g/1 lb	**sweet, ripe seedless grapes**
1 sachet/1 tbs	**gelatine crystals**
½	**lemon, juice of**
½	**orange, juice of**
	sugar to taste

1 Wash the grapes and set aside the best 6 for decoration.
2 Put the rest of the grapes into a liquidizer and blend. Add enough water to make 425ml (¾ pint) liquid.
3 Dissolve the gelatine in 2 tablespoons of hot water and add to the grape purée.
4 Pour into a small saucepan and stir in the lemon and orange juices with sugar to taste.
5 Pour into a serving dish and leave to cool, then place in the fridge to set. Decorate with the reserved grapes, halved, before serving.

fruit and nut crunch

This recipe can be varied in several ways. Any kind of stewed fruit can be used, provided it is not too watery (e.g. rhubarb would be too liquid). Try apple, pear, peach, cherries, or mixtures such as blackberry and apple. Fresh fruit can also be used – pineapple, fresh ripe peach, strawberries, raspberries or any such mixture. Banana can also be used, cut into thin slices and with a little orange juice poured over to moisten it. Any chopped and roasted nuts can be used such as almonds and walnuts. If you cannot buy these already roasted, chop and then dry out in a very low oven for about 20 minutes. If in a hurry put under a medium grill for about 10 minutes.

serves two

1 generous knob	**milk-free, wheat-free margarine**
1 slice	**wheat-free bread, made into crumbs**
3 tsp	**sugar**
1 tbs	**hazelnuts, chopped and roasted**
1 portion	**stewed apricots**

1 Melt the margarine in a small frying pan (skillet).
2 Add the breadcrumbs and fry until golden and crisp.
3 Leave to cool and then stir in the sugar and nuts.
4 Put a layer of the fruit in a large wine glass.
5 Sprinkle with a layer of the crunch mixture.
6 Spoon on another layer of the fruit, using it all up.
7 Finish with the rest of the crunch mixture and flatten.

note to cooks   Although this sweet is crunchiest served cold, it can be served hot too. (Both the crunch and the fruit should be hot.)

breadcrumbs

Wheat-free bread can be made into crumbs quite easily. Cut thick slices and break into pieces. Put into an electric coffee grinder and give them a quick whizz.

stuffed peaches

This makes a nice treat for a special dieter and can be baked in the oven when other items are being baked for the rest of the family, or when special wheat-free bread is being baked on the same setting. A delicious way of using the not-so ripe peaches available from the fruiterer and supermarket.

serves one

1 large	**firm peach**
25g/1oz/1 heaped tbs	**wheat-free crumbs made from sponge buns**
	(see page 170)
3 tsp	**sugar**
1 heaped tsp	**ground almonds**
3 heaped tsp	**milk-free, wheat-free margarine**
sprinkle	**grated lemon rind**
	flaked almonds to decorate

1 Preheat oven to 350°F/180°C/gas mark 4.
2 Wash the peach and remove stone. Scoop a little flesh from around the centre and put into a cup.
3 Add the crumbs, sugar, ground almonds, margarine and lemon rind. Beat to a cream with a small spoon. If the mixture is too stiff add a little water.
4 Divide between the two peach halves and stuff the cavity left by the stone.
5 Put into a small oven-proof dish, greased with milk-free margarine. Sprinkle with flaked almonds.
6 Bake above centre of oven for about 25 to 30 minutes.
7 Serve hot or cold.

red fruit salad

Combine raspberries, strawberries, redcurrants, cherries and blackberries in a dish, as available. Sprinkle with lemon juice and sugar to taste.

oat and raisin pudding

serves two

	sunflower oil for greasing
25g/1oz/¼ cup	**rolled oats**
1 tbs	**brown sugar**
1 heaped tsp	**ground almonds or cashews**
½ small	**lemon, grated rind of**
1 heaped tbs	**raisins**
300ml/½ pint/1¼ cups	**soya milk**

1   Preheat the oven to 325°F/160°C/gas mark 3.
2   Grease a small pie dish and put in the oats, sugar, ground nuts, lemon rind and raisins.
3   Pour the soya milk over and stir.
4   Bake for up to 2 hours, stirring occasionally. Serve hot.

note to cooks   Soya milk (or soya drink) is a good substitute for cow's milk. Buy it at health-food stores or large supermarkets and make sure you get the plain, unflavoured kind (check the label).

baked fruit

Fruit which has been baked in the oven tastes quite different from stewed fruit. Often, if the oven is already being used for another dish, it is easy to put in a dish of fruit to bake. If the oven is on a high heat, put the fruit low down in the oven. If on a medium heat, use the top of the oven.

Several kinds of fruit are suitable for baking – apples, rhubarb, apricots, peaches, plums, greengages, redcurrants and blackcurrants, pears etc., or any mixture in season such as blackberry and apple. Fruit juice, water or wine can be used to keep the fruit moist. Here is a typical example of baked fruit:

baked apricots

1 Put 675g (1½ lb) of fresh, washed apricots, in an ovenproof dish.
2 Sprinkle with sugar to taste and the juice of a lemon. Put on the lid.
3 Bake in a preheated oven at 300°F/150°C/gas mark 2 for about ¾ hour to 1 hour or until the fruit is soft.
4 Serve hot or cold.

baked apples

If baking apples, leave the peel on but remove the central core. Cut a line round the 'waist'. Fill the centre with raisins or other fruit such as raspberries or blackberries. Sprinkle with a little sugar (or liquid honey) and bake in a dish with a little water until soft. This should take about half an hour at 350°F/180°C/gas mark 4. (No lid required.)

pears in wine

Pears can be peeled and left whole. Cooked in red wine with a few pinches of cinnamon, they make a delicious dessert.

baked bananas

Bananas require little cooking time and are best cooked in pineapple or orange juice. Bake in a shallow dish at 350°F/180°C/gas mark 4 for a mere 15 minutes, top shelf. They can be sprinkled with chopped dates instead of a sweetener for variation. (No lid required.)

fruit dessert

1 slightly heaped tbs	**ground brown rice**
150ml/¼ pint/⅔ cup	**unsweetened orange or pineapple juice**
1 tbs	**sugar**
1 tsp	**vegetable oil**

1 Put all ingredients into a small saucepan and mix until smooth.

2 Heat to boiling point and cook, while stirring, for 2 minutes or until thick.

3 Leave to grow cold. Serve chilled from the fridge.

rice and sultana pudding

1 tbs	**soya/soy flour**
½ litre/1 pint/2½ cups	**water**
25g/1oz/2½ tbs	**milk-free margarine**
3 tbs	**brown rice (uncooked)**
2 tbs	**sugar**
1 heaped tbs	**sultanas/golden seedless raisins**
few drops	**pure vanilla flavouring**
	grated nutmeg

1   Put the soya (soy) flour into a saucepan with a little of the water and mix until smooth.
2   Add the rest of the water and bring to the boil. Simmer for 5 minutes.
3   Add the margarine and stir until melted.
4   Put the rice and sugar into an ovenproof dish and pour the soya mixture over it.
5   Add the sultanas (golden seedless raisins) and vanilla flavouring. Stir well.
6   Sprinkle a little nutmeg over the top and bake for about 2½ hours at 275°F/140°C/ gas mark 1. If it starts to dry out during cooking, add a little more (hot) water.

'cheese' and biscuits

For people on a milk-free diet, cheese is definitely out. However, the following recipe has a pleasant cheesy taste and looks very much like cheese spread.

4 tsp	**sunflower oil**
3 pinches	**sea salt**
½	**clove garlic, peeled**
25g/1oz/¼ cup	**ground almonds**
about 8 drops	**fresh lemon juice**

1 Put the oil and salt into a small basin.
2 Rub the cut part of the garlic clove round the basin, spreading the oil and salt. Discard the clove.
3 Put in the ground almonds and mix with a fork to absorb the oil.
4 Add the lemon juice and mix to a paste.
5 Use as a spread on special wheat-free crispbreads or special wheat-free toast.
6 Serve with a crisp eating apple, pear, peach or nectarine and wheat-free crispbreads.

pineapple water ice

A light refreshing sweet that can be stored in the freezer and used as required.

serves four

1 small	**pineapple**
240ml/8oz/1⅓ cups	**water**
1 tbs	**lemon juice**
	sugar to taste

1 Cut off the top and bottom of the pineapple. Trim off outside casing all round and discard. Also cut out the core and discard.
2 Cut flesh into dice and put into a saucepan with the water and lemon juice.
3 Bring to the boil and cook for about 5 minutes, adding sugar to taste.
4 Allow to cool a little and then blend in a liquidizer.
5 Spoon into a freezer container and freeze. Remove from freezer and then beat until the mixture becomes fluffy.
6 Freeze until needed.

apricot and honey dessert

This turns out as quite a creamy sweet yet no milk or cream are used.

serves three

100g/4oz/¾ cup	**dried apricots**
¼	**lemon, juice of**
½	**lemon, rind of**
1½ tbs	**liquid honey**
7g/¼oz	**gelatine crystals**
2 tbs	**water (cold)**

1 Soak the apricots overnight in plenty of cold water.
2 The following day cook in a saucepan with enough water to cover. Bring to the boil and then simmer gently for 30 minutes or until the fruit is soft enough to purée.
3 Put the gelatine and water into a small basin over a pan of simmering water. Stir until dissolved and then mix in well with the apricots.
4 Put the apricots, lemon juice and rind into the blender with the honey. Liquidize.
5 Spoon into 3 glass dishes and leave to cool. Chill in the fridge until set.
6 Serve cold from the fridge.

soya milk pudding

serves four

40g/1½oz/⅓ cup	sago, tapioca, flaked rice or ground rice
1 heaped tbs	brown sugar
pinch	salt
3 pinches	freshly grated nutmeg
2 tsp	sunflower oil
600ml/1 pint/2½ cups	plain, unflavoured soya milk

1 Preheat the oven to 300°F/150°C/gas mark 2.
2 Sprinkle the sago, tapioca or rice into an ovenproof dish with the sugar, salt and nutmeg, then pour in the oil and soya milk.
3 Bake above the centre of the oven for 2½ to 3 hours. Serve hot with stewed, fresh or dried fruit.

note to cooks The grated rind of half a lemon or orange can be substituted for the nutmeg. Instead of the almonds, wheat/milk-free margarine can be used.

teas and treats

It is amazing how many people believe that a 'treat' to someone on a special diet means the very things they are normally not allowed to eat, forgetting that these things will probably cause that person to be ill. The majority of people think that diets are merely for slimming and many are under the illusion that any kind of special diet is just a silly fad.

A treat should be either a special dish or food that is not a normal part of the diet, either because it requires some trouble to make or is expensive. It can also be something seasonal such as mince pies or Christmas cake. Whatever form it takes, it should still be firmly within the confines of the permitted foods on the diet. (*See the index for suggestions.*)

teabread

makes one small loaf

½	medium cooking apple, peeled, cored and sliced thinly
½ cup	water
120g/4oz/⅔ cup	ground rice
60g/2oz/½ cup	barley flour
30g/1oz	oat flour *(see opposite)*
pinch	salt
1 heaped tbs	brown sugar
7g/¼oz	instant yeast
1 tbs	sunflower oil
185ml/6½fl oz/¾ cup	lukewarm tea (without milk)
	finely grated rind of 1 orange
60g/2oz/½ cup	sultanas/golden seedless raisins or raisins, chopped

1 Stew the apple with the ½ cup of water for a few minutes in a small pan. Use a wooden spoon to beat to a smooth purée as soon as it has softened and broken up. Put aside to cool.

2 Preheat oven to 350°F/180°C/gas mark 4.

3 Grease a 500g/1lb loaf tin.

4 Put the flours, salt, sugar, yeast, oil and tea into a bowl. Mix well.

5 Add 3 tbs of the apple purée and mix to a thick, creamy batter with the tea.

6 Stir in the fruit and rind.

7 Turn into the prepared tin and immediately put into the oven on the top shelf to bake for about 1 hour. It will rise and have a cracked top.

8 As soon as it looks golden, turn out of the tin and leave to cool on a wire rack. Do not cut until cold as it needs to 'set', and avoid squeezing the loaf as this will cause it to crack inside.

9 Eat freshly baked for tea or for a snack. Slice thickly and spread with milk-free margarine. The following day eat toasted.

note to cooks   As soon as the loaf has cooled down, wrap in food film to prevent drying out. Grind porridge oats in a coffee grinder (electric) to make oat flour.

spicy currant bread

Make as for teabread but omit raisins or sultanas. Instead, use currants and ½ level teaspoon mixed spice.

walnut loaf

Make as for Teabread but omit raisins or sultanas. Instead, use chopped walnuts, toasted under the grill on a baking sheet until lightly browned. A generous tablespoon of thick honey can be used instead of the brown sugar. For extra walnut flavour, instead of 1 tablespoon of sunflower oil use 2 teaspoons of walnut oil and 2 teaspoons of sunflower oil. (Buy the walnut oil at supermarkets.)

note to cooks   Although this loaf contains yeast it does not need to be left to rise. No kneading is required as the mixture is a kind of batter. The loaf will rise by about 50 per cent during baking and should be brown and crusty.

Use for snacks or for tea sliced thickly and spread with milk-free margarine. Also good toasted the day after baking.

fruit and nut cookies

makes ten

50g/2oz/¼ cup	**polyunsaturated wheat-free, milk-free margarine**
75g/3oz/¾ cup	**ground rice**
25g/1oz/¼ cup	**ground almonds**
75g/3oz/¾ cup	**eating apple, finely grated**
½ tsp	**cinnamon**
40g/1½oz/3 tbs	**soft brown (molasses) sugar, plus extra for sprinkling**
few drops	**almond flavouring**
½	**lemon, grated rind of**
50g/2oz/⅓ cup	**mixed dried fruit**
	sunflower oil for greasing

1 Preheat the oven to 450°F/230°C/gas mark 8.
2 Put all the ingredients except the sunflower oil in a bowl and mix together with a wooden spoon to form a dough.
3 Grease a baking (cookie) sheet with sunflower oil. Divide the dough into 10 pieces and arrange them on the baking (cookie) sheet, spreading them out with a knife. Sprinkle with sugar.
4 Bake for about 20 minutes, until golden. Leave on the baking (cookie) sheet to cool for 10 minutes, then transfer to a wire rack with a spatula. Eat within 2 days.

carob cake

25g/1oz/¾ cup	**soya/soy flour**
50g/3oz/½ cup	**sugar**
1½ tbs	**home-made pectin**
25g/1oz/¼ cup	**wheat-free carob powder**
75g/3oz/½ cup	**ground brown rice**
50g/2oz/½ cup	**barley flour**
25g/1oz/½ cup	**finely ground nuts**
2 heaped tsp	**special wheat-free and milk-free baking powder** *(see page 29)*
150ml/¼ pint/⅔ cup	**orange juice**
75g/3oz/1 small	**finely grated apple**
2 tbs	**sunflower oil**

1 Preheat oven to 400°F/200°C/gas mark 6.
2 Put all the ingredients into a bowl and mix to a cream.
3 Grease a tin size 185 x 90 x 60mm (7¼ x 3½ x 2¼ inches). Use milk-free margarine or sunflower oil. 'Flour' with ground rice.
4 Spoon in the mixture and flatten with a knife.
5 Bake on the top shelf for about 45 to 50 minutes.
6 Turn out onto a wire rack to cool.
7 When quite cold, store in a sealed plastic bag.
8 Eat within 2 or 3 days.

note to cooks   Use only home-made pectin and not the commercial type used for making jams. Most of the work in this recipe is in the weighing out, which should be accurate and not guessed.

chocolate cake

Use the Carob Cake recipe but substitute wheat-free cocoa powder for the carob.

ginger cake

Use the Carob Cake recipe but instead of carob add 2 heaped teaspoonsful ground ginger.

party almonds

Spread shelled almonds in a shallow baking tin and toast in a preheated oven to 350°F/180°C/gas mark 4 for about 6 minutes on the top shelf. Serve cold as a party nibble.

fruit salad cake

7g/¼oz/1 tbs	Easyblend (instant) dried yeast
25g/1oz/¼ cup	soya/soy flour
160g/6oz/1½ cups	ground rice
25g/1oz/¼ cup	wheat-free cornflour/(cornstarch)
50g/2oz/½ cup	ground almonds
75g/3oz/⅓ cup	brown sugar, plus extra for sprinkling
2 tsp	cinnamon
3 tbs	sunflower oil
150ml/¼ pint	pineapple juice
1 medium	eating apple, cored and sliced (do not peel)
50g/2oz	carrot, sliced
1	lemon, grated rind of
225g/8oz/1⅓ cups	dried fruit salad, such as prunes, apricots, peaches, pears, chopped
	sunflower oil for greasing

1   Preheat the oven to 350°F/180°C/gas mark 4.

2   Mix the yeast, soya (soy) flour, ground almonds, sugar and cinnamon in a bowl, then stir in the oil.

3   Warm the pineapple juice to lukewarm in a small pan, then pour into a liquidizer. Add the apple and carrot and blend to a purée. Pour into the flour mixture and stir well.

4   Stir in the chopped dried fruit and turn into a greased soufflé dish. Smooth the top with a knife and sprinkle with sugar.

5   Bake above the centre of the oven for about an hour or until a skewer inserted in the centre comes out clean.

6   Leave to cool in the dish before turning out. Store wrapped in the fridge and eat within a week.

apple and sultana flapjacks

	sunflower oil or margarine for greasing
1 medium	cooking apple, peeled, cored and coarsely grated
1 heaped tbs	sultanas/golden seedless raisins
90g/3½oz/½ cup	soft brown/molasses sugar
100g/4oz/½ cup	wheat-free, milk-free margarine
40g/1½oz/⅓ cup	ground rice mixed with ½ tsp wheat-free baking powder
100g/4oz/2 cups	rolled oats

1 Preheat the oven to 350°F/180°C/gas mark 4. Grease the base of a square 15cm (6 inch) cake tin (cake pan) with oil or margarine.

2 Put the grated apple, sultanas (golden seedless raisins) and 1 tablespoon of the sugar into a small pan. Heat gently for 5 minutes, stirring, until the mixture is soft and the sultanas plump.

3 In a separate pan, melt the margarine over a low heat. Take off the heat and stir in the ground rice and baking powder mixture with the remaining sugar and oats.

4 Spread half the oat mixture over the base of the tin, pressing it down with the back of a spoon. Spread the apple filling evenly over the top.

5 Top with the remaining oat mixture, sprinkling it on and pressing down firmly.

6 Bake at the top of the oven for 30 to 35 minutes, until golden. Cool in the tin (pan) and cut into 16 small squares. Store in an airtight container and eat within 4 days.

date and ginger cake

7g/¼oz/1 tbs	Easyblend (instant) yeast
25g/1oz/¼ cup	soya/soy flour (low fat)
200g/7oz/1½ cups	ground rice
50g/2oz/¼ cup	brown sugar
1 tsp	ground ginger
150ml/¼ pint/⅔ cup	orange juice
65g/2½oz/5 tbs	polyunsaturated wheat-free, milk-free margarine
1	eating apple, cored and sliced (do not peel)
50g/2oz	carrot, sliced
225g/8oz/1¼ cups	stoned chopped dates

1 Preheat the oven to 350°F/180°C/gas mark 4.

2 Mix the yeast, soya (soy) flour, ground rice, ground almonds, sugar and ginger together in a bowl.

3 Put the fruit juice and margarine in a pan and heat to lukewarm. Pour into the flour mixture.

4 Put the apple and carrot in a liquidizer with the fruit juice. Blend and pour into the bowl. Mix well.

5 Stir in the dates and turn into a greased soufflé dish. Smooth the top with a knife.

6 Bake for about 1 hour or until a skewer inserted in the centre comes out clean. Leave to cool in the dish before turning out. Store wrapped in the fridge and eat within 1 week.

apricot and cinnamon cake

Make as for Date and Ginger Cake but substitute dried apricots and cinnamon for the dates and ginger.

sweet mincemeat

75g/3oz/½ cup	sultanas/golden seedless raisins
50g/2oz/⅓ cup	raisins
75g/3oz/½ cup	currants
50g/2oz/⅓ cup	sugar
50g/2oz/¼ cup	melted milk-free margarine
50g/2oz/½ cup	chopped walnuts/English walnuts and almonds mixed
½ tsp	allspice
½ tsp	cinnamon
½ tsp	freshly grated nutmeg
1	lemon, finely grated rind of
1	eating apple, grated
	orange juice, fresh

1 Blend all ingredients in a bowl and moisten with a little orange juice – about 2 tablespoonsful should be enough.
2 Store in covered jars in the fridge and use as required.

note to cooks   This will keep for several weeks. As the commercial type of sweet mincemeat usually contains suet, which is rolled in wheat flour, home-made mincemeat will be the safest to use and is really much nicer than the bought kind.

Use to stuff baked apples.

rich fruit and nut cake

This is a lovely, rich and moist cake, indistinguishable from the kind made with wheat flour, butter and eggs. It is a good cake to serve for Christmas and birthdays.

7g/¼oz/1 tbs	**Easyblend (instant) yeast (milk-free brand)**
2½ tbs	**sunflower oil**
150ml/¼ pint/⅔ cup	**pineapple juice**
75g/3oz/¾ cup	**eating apple, cored and chopped (do not peel)**
40g/1½oz/½ cup	**carrot, sliced**
few drops	**almond flavouring**
225g/8oz/1⅓ cups	**dried mixed fruit, washed**
50g/2oz/⅓ cup	**glacé/candied cherries, washed**
2 small	**lemons, grated rind of**
	split almonds, walnut halves, cashews, pecan nuts or any kind of plain nuts to decorate

flour blend:

2 heaped tbs	**soft brown/molasses sugar**
125g/5oz/1¼ cups	**ground rice**
25g/1oz/¼ cup	**soya/soy flour**
2 tsp	**cinnamon**
2 tsp	**wheat-free mixed spice**
¼ tsp	**ground nutmeg**
50g/2oz/½ cup	**ground almonds**

1   Preheat the oven to 350°F/180°C/gas mark 4.

2   Put all the ingredients for the flour blend in a bowl and mix well. Sprinkle in the yeast and oil and stir to combine.

3   Warm the pineapple juice to lukewarm in a small pan. Pour into a liquidizer, add the apple and carrot pieces and blend.

4   Pour into the flour mixture and stir well.

5   Add the dried fruit and cherries. Mix well and then spoon into a 15 to 18cm (6 to 7 inch) cake tin (cake pan) that has been oiled with sunflower oil. Smooth the top and lightly press in the nuts in circles.

6   Bake for an hour on the top shelf of the oven, until a skewer inserted in the centre comes out clean. Leave to cool in the tin (pan) before turning out.

7   Store wrapped in greaseproof (wax) paper in the fridge and eat within a week.

sponge buns

makes five

3 level tbs	**apple purée** *(see below)*
45g/1½oz	**caster sugar**
45g/1½oz	**ground rice**
15g/½oz	**cornflour (cornstarch)**
15g/½oz	**barley flour**
2 tbs	**sunflower oil**
¼ tsp	**vanilla flavouring**

1 Preheat oven to 350°F/180°C/gas mark 4.

2 Put all ingredients into a bowl. Stir/beat to a smooth, thick and creamy batter.

3 Have ready a patty tin lined with 5 cake papers.

4 Bake for 20 minutes on the top shelf. Put onto a wire rack to cool.

5 Eat freshly baked. When cold they can be wrapped individually in food film for the following day. Use to make trifle if there are any left over.

note to cooks   To make apple purée, peel and core 1 small cooking apple. Slice thinly and put into a small saucepan with enough water to cover. Cook over a medium heat until the apple has softened and starts to break up. Continue to cook while stirring until you have a smooth purée.

lemon buns

Make as for Sponge Buns but omit vanilla and add the finely grated rind of ¼ lemon.

orange buns

Make as for Sponge Buns but omit vanilla and add the finely grated rind of ⅓ orange.

chocolate buns

Make as for Sponge Buns but add 1 heaped tsp cocoa powder (wheat-free). If the mixture turns out too stiff, add 2 tsp water and mix again.

sultana scones

makes six small scones

30g/1oz	**oat flour**
30g/1oz	**cornflour**
115g/4oz/⅔ cup	**ground rice**
¼ level tsp	**bicarbonate of soda**
½ level tsp	**cream of tartar**
1 slightly rounded tbs	**caster sugar**
30g/1oz	**milk-free margarine**
60g/2oz/⅔ cup	**fresh mashed potato**
60g/2oz/½ cup	**sultanas, chopped**
	soya milk or water, to bind

1 Preheat oven to 425°F/220°C/gas mark 7.

2 Mix the first six (dry) ingredients in a bowl.

3 Rub in the margarine and then the potato.

4 Sprinkle in the fruit.

5 Stir in enough soya milk to bind and mix to a smooth, stiff dough. Divide into 6 pieces and shape each one into a scone.

6 Put onto a greased baking sheet and bake for 15 minutes on the top shelf.

7 When golden brown, cool on a wire rack.

8 Serve split and spread with milk-free margarine. Eat freshly baked. Any left over can be individually wrapped in food film and split and toasted the following day.

note to cooks   To make oat flour, grind porridge oats in a coffee grinder (electric).

apple chutney

½ kilo/1 lb	**cooking apples, peeled and chopped**
100g/4oz/1 cup	**onions, peeled and chopped**
75g/3oz/½ cup	**sultanas/golden seedless raisins**
150ml/¼ pint/⅔ cup	**cider vinegar**
50g/2oz/⅓ cup	**sugar**
¼ tsp	**ground ginger**
¼ tsp	**sea salt**

1 Cook the apple, onion, sultanas (golden seedless raisins) and dates in the vinegar until soft.
2 Add the remaining ingredients and stir well.
3 Bring to the boil and simmer until you have a thick chutney.
4 Put into clean, hot jars and allow to cool before covering.
5 Store in the fridge and use as required. (Serve with curry or cold meats.)

tomato ketchup

½ kilo/1 lb	**ripe tomatoes**
3 tsp	**tarragon wine vinegar**
3 tbs	**sugar**
2 pinches	**each of cinnamon, cayenne pepper, sea salt, ground mace and allspice**

1　Put the tomatoes into a pan, after slicing. Add a little water if required and cook for about 3 or 4 minutes, while stirring.
2　Allow to cool and liquidize.
3　Return to pan and add sugar and spices. Stir well.
4　Bring to the boil and simmer until it has reduced to a thick sauce.
5　Allow to grow cold and put into a sauce bottle or jar. Use as required. Best stored in the fridge.

wheat, milk
and egg-free menus

Each day drink tea with lemon or black coffee, water or wine with your main meal if desired. Tea (food) is optional.

suggestions for meals

breakfasts

Savoury Breakfast Cakes with grilled tomatoes.

Small Muesli, grilled bacon and tomatoes.

Grilled bacon, tomatoes, fried mushrooms, special toast, milk-free margarine and raw sugar marmalade.

Breakfast Pizza.

Grilled fish, tomatoes and crispbreads with milk-free margarine.

Fruit pancakes or Granola, cold meat.

Grapefruit, slice of cold ham, tomato, special bread or crispbreads, milk-free margarine.

Fried potato and baked beans with mushrooms.

Baked beans on special toast with tomatoes.

Bubble and Squeak with grilled bacon, special toast, milk-free margarine and raw sugar
marmalade.

Grapefruit with sugar, Kedgeree.

Savoury Breakfast Cakes, Fruit Pancake.

(Tea with lemon or black coffee, fruit juice, as required.)

light meals (suitable for lunch or high tea)

Fish Cakes with mixed salad.

Cold meat or fish with salad and mashed potato.

Liver and Mushroom Pâté on special toast with green salad.

French Country Soup with Sippets, Fruit Tart with Nuts.

Lentil Soup, jacket potato stuffed with chopped grilled bacon and mushrooms.

Shepherd's Pie with peas and grilled tomatoes.

Fish and chips with peas or grilled tomatoes.

main meals

Prawns Italian with green salad, plain boiled brown rice.

Lemon Chicken, plain boiled brown rice, green salad or stir-fry vegetables with plenty of
green leaves.

Shepherd's Pie, carrots, peas, cabbage or sprouts.

Liver Provençale with plain boiled brown rice or mashed potatoes, green vegetables.

Goulash with plain boiled brown rice, green salad.

Roast beef or lamb (joint) with roast potatoes, green vegetables in season, special
gravy.

Pork Chop with Apple Salad, jacket potato.

Trout with Almonds, peas or a mixed salad.

Grilled Fish with Herbs, peas and carrots.

Lamb with Garlic and Rosemary (chops), roast potatoes and parsnip, greens.

Kebabs with plain boiled brown rice, green salad.

Baked Trout with mashed potato, grilled tomatoes, peas.

Grilled Steak with spinach, carrots and grilled tomatoes or Savoury Rice *(see page 133)*.

Grilled lamb chops (plain) with Savoury Rice.

Chicken Curry with plain boiled brown rice, sliced cucumber and banana; Poppadoms.

Chicken and Herb Casserole, mashed or jacket potato, green vegetables.

Beef Casserole with Orange, stir-fry vegetables.

Good, Old Fashioned Stew with green vegetables.

Lemon Chicken and Chinese Fried Rice, stir-fry vegetables.

Bolognese Sauce with plain boiled brown rice, green salad.

Nut Roast, green vegetables, mashed potato.

Combine any of these main meals with a recipe from the puddings section to make a substantial meal. Really hearty eaters will enjoy something from the section which contains soups and starters too.

teas

The bread-and-butter and cake teas our grandparents enjoyed have largely gone out of fashion. However, youngsters often go through a stage of always feeling hungry, usually when they are growing very quickly (early teens), and this can be a useful way of giving them an extra meal without too much trouble. Tea-time is also a good opportunity to use up any kind of pudding left from the previous day.

Slice of fruit cake (from *Teas and Treats* section), apple.

Slices of Tea Bread or Currant Bread with milk-free, wheat-free margarine, fruit cake
(from *Teas and Treats* section), banana.

Special toast, milk-free, wheat-free margarine and jam (jelly), nuts.

Crispbreads and milk-free, wheat-free margarine.

Soup with Sippets, fruit cake (from *Teas and Treats* section).

useful information

general items

Available at most supermarkets or grocery stores and health stores:

Ground rice	Fruit juices
Spices	Wine or cider vinegar
Sunflower and olive oils	(not malt)
Easyblend (instant) yeast	Porridge oats
(check ingredients for	Milk-free, wheat-free
milk derivatives)	margarine (non-dairy)
Pure cornflour (cornstarch)	

specialized items

Probably available at health stores, delicatessens or large chemists (drugstores):

Soya flour	Millet flour
Potato flour (farina)	(Gram) chickpea flour
Barley and rye flours	Tamari-type wheat-free
Oatmeal	soy/soya sauce

fan ovens – temperature and baking times

As these may vary from one model to another, only guidelines can be given. Generally speaking, temperatures of 20° below those recommended for an ordinary oven and baking times of up to one third less should be effective.

index